OXFORD MEDICAL PUBLICATIONS

Accidents and Emergencies

Accidents and Emergencies

A PRACTICAL HANDBOOK
FOR PERSONAL USE

R. H. HARDY

Formerly Consultant in Accident and Emergency Medicine
Hereford General Hospital

Fifth edition

Revised by

John Bache

Consultant in Accident and Emergency Medicine
Leighton Hospital
Crewe

OXFORD NEW YORK TOKYO
OXFORD UNIVERSITY PRESS
1987

Oxford University Press, Walton Street, Oxford OX2 6DP

Oxford New York Toronto
Delhi Bombay Calcutta Madras Karachi
Petaling Jaya Singapore Hong Kong Tokyo
Nairobi Dar es Salaam Cape Town
Melbourne Auckland

and associated companies in
Beirut Berlin Ibadan Nicosia

Oxford is a trade mark of Oxford University Press

Published in the United States
by Oxford University Press, New York

First edition published 1976 by Robert Dugdale
Second edition published 1978 by Oxford University Press
Third edition 1981
Fourth edition 1985
Fifth edition 1987

British Library Cataloguing in Publication Data
Hardy, R. H.
Accidents and emergencies: a practical
handbook for personal use.—5th ed.—
(Oxford medical publications).
1. Emergency medicine
I. Title   II. Bache, John B.
616'.025   RC86.7
ISBN 0–19–261650–1

Library of Congress Cataloging in Publication Data
Hardy, R. H.
Accidents and emergencies.
(Oxford medical publications)
Bibliography: p.
Includes index.
1. Emergency medicine—Handbooks, manuals, etc.
2. Accidents—Handbooks, manuals, etc.   I. Bache, John B.
II. Title.   III. Series. [DNLM: 1. Accidents—handbooks.
2. Emergencies—handbooks.   3. First Aid—Handbooks.
WA 39 H271a]
RC86.8.H37 1987   616'.025   87–12277
ISBN 0–19–261650–1 (pbk.)

Set by Cotswold Typesetting Ltd, Cheltenham
Printed in Great Britain
at the University Printing House, Oxford
by David Stanford
Printer to the University

Preface to the fifth edition

The sense of honour I felt when I was invited to assume responsibility for Richard Hardy's book was tempered with trepidation. The success of the previous four editions was indicative of its worth. Therefore to change it was to invite criticism.

It was, I felt, imperative to retain the original intention of the book, which was to provide practical advice for the casualty officer facing unfamiliar situations and expected to make immediate decisions. However, a number of new sections were needed, such as one on cot death and a few words about some common mistakes; other sections required lengthening. Yet the length of the book itself had to be kept within strict limits and alternate pages remain blank for the owner's personal comments, as was Dr Hardy's original intention. The net result was that some sections had to be radically shortened or even omitted altogether. I tried to make these cuts in those places where information, interesting as it may have been, was unlikely to be urgently required by a casualty officer, or was easily accessible elsewhere, from standard texts. Topics such as pyrexia of unknown origin, infestation, gas gangrene, etc., have thus been radically shortened. Every Accident and Emergency department must have a small library to provide urgently needed information, and this assumption allowed me to omit other sections, such as drug doses: the most meagrely equipped department must surely possess a *British National Formulary* and a *Data Sheet Compendium*. Some rather obscure entries, such as proctalgia fugax and yaws, have also disappeared.

So far as fractures are concerned, previous editions have received some adverse criticism. There are a number of excellent books devoted to fractures and it is not my intention to compete with them. On the other hand, certain fractures and dislocations are of particular importance to the casualty officer and I have therefore placed emphasis on these, for example Colles' fracture, pulled elbow, dislocation of the shoulder, etc. The resulting balance is, as always, open to criticism.

I have included a number of new references, mostly

from the *British Medical Journal*, so that the interested casualty officer will have easy access to them.

Accident and emergency medicine has no equal in terms of its variety, excitement, stress, and the proportion of patients who fully recover. It is the oldest branch of medicine. It is very rewarding. But it is full of potential problems. If this book improves your personal safety record, it will be a success.

Crewe,   J.B.B.
January 1987

Preface to the first edition

I have found a continual need of a handbook to give to medical and nursing staff coming to accident and emergency work for the first time, and I know that many others in my place have found the same.

This one is based on the handbook which grew up in Hereford, but it has been largely rewritten after the critical scrutiny of many friends and colleagues, in particular Mr James Scott, FRCS, who has gone through the text with a thoroughness that I cannot thank him enough for, and Miss Sheila Christian, FRCS, who has made many useful suggestions and criticisms.

Any textbook of accidents and emergencies will have limitations because of the lack of any generally accepted practice in the field, the absence of any received dogma, and the fact that all medical and surgical practice is in a state of flux. Besides which, the variations between different parts of the country and different hospitals make any definitive textbook of little value except as a basic source book. So the solution is offered here of a skeleton text upon which the casualty officer can build his own code with the help of his seniors in the special fields of accidents and emergencies, orthopaedics, and all the other specialities which overlap with them.

The opinions and guidance offered are often heterodox and sometimes frankly contentious in the hope that they may stimulate radical rethinking of current practice and a revaluation of every user's concepts in the light of his own experience as well as ours. The text on the left-hand page is only a framework upon which the reader can build. What will be really valuable is what is written on the right.

Accident and emergency work is emerging as a career which attracts more medical talent each year because of the increasing realization of its capacity for growth and improvement in giving help to the injured and acutely ill, and the endless opportunity and interest it offers to its practitioners as its scope and skill develop. This very tentative compilation is made in the hope that beginners of all sorts may find it a useful basis for building up their own expertise.

A casualty officer in the medical organism has been compared to the hand in the individual's constitution—both are the most highly unspecialized organs in the body. So the keynote of a book designed to help the first to be fully effective has to be adaptable versatility.

My thanks to my publisher, Robert Dugdale, are limitless for his faith in my undertaking and for the endless pains he has taken in trying to make a silk purse out of a sow's ear. I have been continually helped and encouraged by his critical enthusiasm and hope that he will have no occasion to regret his daring.

Needless to say the responsibility for everything written here is my own, but it would unquestionably have been far worse without the help of all the many people who have been so generous with their aid.

R.H.H.

Acknowledgements

Authors and publisher would like to thank Smith and Nephew Pharmaceuticals for Figs 2 and 3.

John Bache is sincerely grateful to Dr John McKay (Consultant Physician), Dr Robert Pugh (Consultant Paediatrician), Miss Pauline Leaver (Consultant Obstetrician and Gynaecologist), and Dr Howard Allison (Consultant Pathologist) for their valued criticism of the relevant sections of the text.

Note: Although much of Dr Hardy's text survives unchanged in this edition, responsibility for the content of the book is now borne solely by Mr Bache.

Note: Arrangement of the text

The text is arranged alphabetically by subject (there is also a detailed index at the back of the book). Main entries are marked ■. Right-hand pages have been left blank for the reader's own notes, additions, and updates.

**To Lorraine
Sarah
and Pauline**

Contents

While every effort has been made to check drug dosages in this book, it is still possible that errors have been missed. Furthermore, dosage schedules are being continually revised and new side-effects recognized. For these reasons the reader is strongly urged to consult the drug companies' printed instructions before administering any of the drugs recommended in this book.

■ Abdominal injuries

These are common in road traffic accidents, horse-riding accidents, gunshot wounds, stabbings, agricultural accidents, and domestic accidents. Initial management:

1 Establish baseline observations (pulse rate, blood pressure, respiratory rate, girth).
2 Take blood samples for full blood count, urea and electrolytes, amylase, arterial gases, and cross-matching. Test the urine.
3 Establish an intravenous infusion in a good vein (cf. **Shock, surgical**).
4 Arrange X-rays, e.g. erect chest (look for gas under the diaphragm and lower rib fractures), erect and supine abdomen (look for fractures of the transverse processes and obliterated psoas outline), and pelvis.
5 Consider peritoneal lavage, bladder catheterization, nasogastric tube, endotracheal intubation, intravenous pyelography, antibiotics, and tetanus prophylaxis.

Frequent reassessment is mandatory. Rising pulse rate, falling blood pressure, tenderness, guarding, rigidity, absent bowel sounds, increasing abdominal girth, and the return of blood on peritoneal lavage all suggest that laparotomy is necessary.

Bruising of the soft abdominal wall or fabric imprints on to the skin over soft parts are serious signs. Associated low rib fractures alert the examiner to the possibility of splenic or hepatic injury.

If an abdominal injury is one of many, especially if consciousness is lost, it is very easy to miss it. Having estimated the volume of blood loss from the known injuries and given suitable fluids in accordance with the expected needs of the patient, surgical shock may yet persist ('unresponsive hypotension'); this suggests bleeding into the chest (which should be visible on X-ray) or into the abdomen.

In all cases of multiple injuries where there is any risk of abdominal injury as well, girth measurements should

be made at a marked level every 10 minutes and recorded. Increasing girth is a warning of bleeding or ileus.

Left shoulder tip pain suggests a ruptured spleen. A fit young adult with a ruptured spleen can maintain blood pressure and pulse rate at fairly normal levels for some time, giving a false sense of security to the inexperienced, until suddenly the blood loss reaches a level at which the cardiovascular system can no longer cope, so that the patient rapidly goes into dramatic hypovolaemic shock, requiring urgent laparotomy. Ruptured spleens may bleed slowly; they may also develop a subcapsular haematoma which can rupture in 7–15 days.

A ruptured liver is a common event in blunt abdominal trauma and is often only clearly identified at laparotomy.

Traumatic perforation of the bowel usually occurs at a site where external compression meets internal resistance, e.g. where the duodeno-jejunal junction rests on the third lumbar vertebra. Tears of the mesocolon and other mesenteries in the midline can also occur.

Renal damage may arise from direct violence to the loin; pelvic viscera can be involved in injuries to the bony pelvis, notably the bladder and urethra.

In general, early operation is not all that important in stab wounds, but awareness of the possibility of multiple perforations and the likelihood of bowel trauma in the absence of a clear wound-track through the abdominal parietes will make the observer alert to changes in the patient's physical signs.

Peritoneal lavage is often useful: after catheterization of the bladder, use a dialysis catheter introduced through a small incision, suprapubically in the midline, half-way between pubes and umbilicus. One litre of warm normal saline is used for lavage and a two-way tap for drainage into a bottle with underwater seal.

A high index of suspicion in casualty officers is of far more value than special investigations if abdominal injuries are not to be missed.

See also **Stab wounds** and **Urogenital injuries**

■ Abortions

Threatened, inevitable, incomplete, or complete, abortions are unpredictable and often combined with anxiety and fear. They are best dealt with in a specialist unit, and should be given the briefest of examinations and transmitted as soon as possible to their proper destination, unless urgent resuscitation is required on arrival.

Intravenous Syntometrine 1 ml (ergometrine maleate 500 μg + oxytocin 5 U) may control bleeding. Septic abortions should receive intravenous clindamycin 300 mg as well.

Cf. **Obstetric emergencies**

■ Abscesses

Small ones can often be incised under intradermal local anaesthetic, but it is difficult to ensure full breakdown of loculi and proper clearance in big ones. Infected sebaceous cysts respond well. Some authorities dislike local infiltration of abnormal skin but no ill effects have been observed in practice.

Other abscesses are best opened under general anaesthetic. If of any size they are traditionally fully explored by the gloved finger and ribbon gauze inserted to ensure proper drainage. Drainage is prevented by tight packing and this method should now be relegated to history.

Combined drainage and systemic antibiotics give quicker healing than either separately, and should always be used together.

If you don't like the look of it refer it to a senior member of the staff.

Subcuticular abscesses should be *completely* unroofed.

Test the urine of *every* case for sugar.

There are 10 steps:

1 Exclude patients with valvular disease of the heart.
2 Give an intramuscular injection of clindamycin phosphate 300 mg 1 hour pre-operatively.
3 General anaesthesia is desirable.
4 Make an incision of sufficient size to admit one exploring index finger.
5 Explore digitally and drain the pus; send pus for culture and sensitivity.
6 Curette the entire pyogenic membrane and dry the cavity with gauze.
7 Irrigate, without raising the pressure inside the cavity, using hydrogen peroxide solution (20 ml syringe and filling 'quill').
8 Occlude the cavity with deep, encircling, mattress sutures, using a monofilament material.
9 After the first 24 hours, twice daily hot baths are comforting and helpful; topical povidone-iodine ointment after bathing is antiseptic and soothing.
10 The sutures are removed about one week after surgery.

The choice of antibiotic is important: all abscesses below the waist merit treatment with clindamycin, as infections are usually mixed and include anaerobes. An increasing number of other abscesses contain anaerobes as well and the characteristic stink of the pus generally gives them away. If the infection is clearly staphylococcal, flucloxacillin 1 g is given by injection, unless the patient is allergic to penicillin.

A post-operative course of antibiotic appears unnecessary (Blick, P. W. H., Flowers, M. W., Marsden, A. K., Wilson, D. H., and Ghoneim, A. T. M. (1980). Antibiotics in surgical treatment of acute abscesses. *British Medical Journal*, **ii**, 111–12).

The benefit to patients of this out-patient treatment of major abscesses is incalculable: 2 visits (for operation and removal of sutures) instead of dozens; minimal pain and inconvenience, brief recovery period, diminished recurrence. It does a great deal, too, to relieve the pressure of repeated attendances at A & E departments. Traditionalists sometimes cavil, but only those who haven't tried it.

Don't forget: it depends for its success on thorough and complete surgery and the appropriate use of antibiotics; it is *not* suitable for hand infections; it is suitable for *all* other major abscesses.

In my opinion, pilonidal abscesses, ischiorectal abscesses, and perianal abscesses should be treated by the general surgeons, rather than by the casualty officer.

Cf. **Hand infections and injuries**

■ Accidents, major (multiple injuries)

With head, or multiple and head, injuries the routine is simple and must always be followed:

1 Ensure **airway**, with a cuffed tube if necessary, and ventilation — get an anaesthetist fast if in difficulty or doubt.
2 Stop major external **bleeding**, usually by local pressure.
3 Strip and **examine**.
4 Step up **intravenous fluids** if necessary — 4 may need to precede 3 — bilaterally if required and always in the arms if possible, having first taken blood specimens for cross-matching and any relevant baseline estimations. In cases of major or multiple injuries, give steroids.
5 Investigate **injuries**, and record their nature and significance.
6 **Treat** if required.
7 The importance of getting as clear a **history** as possible must not be forgotten, but circumstances may prevent it.
8 A single-shot lateral X-ray of the neck is needed in all unconscious patients.

A central venous pressure (CVP) catheter may be inserted in the A & E department, but this tends to take up time which could be more usefully employed in this vital first hour. Initial management of the patient is determined by his clinical condition, rather than his CVP; leave the CVP until he reaches ITU.

Any major accident demands a combined operation and the more relevant help you get in, after the first assessment of the situation, the better for everyone, especially the patient. Evidence from witnesses and ambulance personnel can be of vital importance in the first assessment.

With practice you should be able to make a reliable assessment of the number and severity of injuries in a 5-minute examination. Your findings should be briefly but clearly recorded, starting at the top, like this:

Part of the body	Injuries
Head and oropharynx	....
Central nervous system	....
Chest	....
Abdomen	....
Pelvis	....
Upper limbs	....
Lower limbs	....
Skin	....
Other	....

One of the few bits of gadgetry which is of real value is an automatic vital-signs monitor. It gives readings of pulse and blood pressure at set intervals and an alarm (pre-set) warns of undue changes.

Intravenous analgesia is the best method of pain relief after trauma; it is of rapid onset but short duration.

Cf. **Pain**

Steroids

All major and multiple injuries should be protected against:

- Fat embolism
- Shock-lung
- Disseminated intravascular coagulation
- Post-traumatic increased capillary permeability

The first and most vital remedy is blood volume replacement, but the role of steroids must not be forgotten. Give 2 g of methylprednisolone intravenously

over 15 minutes. This may be preventative and probably is.

Cf. **Chest injuries**

■ Accidents, road traffic

Injuries are often multiple. It is easy to overlook an associated injury by concentrating on the primary one, e.g.

- In cases of dashboard injury to the knee it is important to X-ray the ipsilateral hip to exclude fracture/dislocation
- In cases of head injury with loss of consciousness it is easy to miss an associated fracture/dislocation of the cervical spine
- Severely injured people are often also drunk (and vice versa)—ask for urgent blood-alcohol levels (if available) to help clarify the severity of their head injuries.

You will quickly adopt your own or your department's techniques for the reception and treatment of such patients. It will not be helpful to write out a scheme here. Make your own, make it infallible, and record it on the opposite page.

■ Actinomycosis

A rare cause of subacute submandibular abscess, likely to be secondary to periodontal infection. Advanced actinomycosis is unheard of today in medically sophisticated countries. Treatment is by surgical drainage and appropriate antibiotics.

■ Adhesives

Cyanoacrylate adhesives have introduced a new dimension into emergency procedure. Their adhesion is instant. A child can stick fingers indissolubly together, gum up his eyes, nose, and mouth with a single smearing gesture and die of suffocation. The manufacturers comfortingly advise peeling apart adherent skin surfaces after applying warm soapy water. Emergency laryngostomy may however be required.

In general, passive non-surgical first aid is all that is needed.

Every accident department should obtain the manufacturer's well-prepared advice-sheet (*Information for first aid and casualty on treatment for adhesion of human skin to itself if caused by cyanoacrylate adhesives*), available on application to Loctite (UK) Ltd, Welwyn Garden City, Herts, AL7 1JB.

■ Anaesthesia, local and regional

Digital nerve block for fingers and toes

If this is done well, it works perfectly. If it is done badly, it is ghastly and saps the patient's confidence like nothing else.

Where appropriate, the injection should be given from the dorsal side into the interdigital web—lignocaine 1% 3–5 ml each side in adults. The needle should point towards the digital nerve (see Fig. 1a,b). If there is no web, local anaesthetic should be injected from the dorsum of the finger until the bulge is palpated in the volar aspect (about 2.5 ml in children, 3–5 ml in adults). Wait 3 minutes.

Do not forget 2 ml of lignocaine 1% across the dorsum of toe or finger to anaesthetize branches of a variable dorsal nerve supply if you wish to operate on the dorsal surface between the base of the digit and the base of the nail.

Never use adrenaline in fingers or toes.

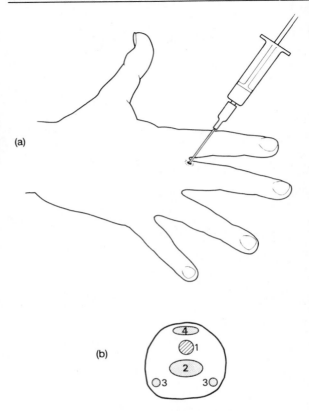

Fig. 1. (a) Position of needle; (b) cross-sectional schema of finger showing position of the digital nerves. 1. phalanx, 2. flexor tendon and fibrous flexor sheath, 3. neuro-vascular bundle, 4. extensor tendon.

Intermetacarpal block

Should always be given from the dorsum of the hand and it is wise to give 8–10 ml of lignocaine 1% either side of the relevant metacarpal.

Bupivacaine 0.5% gives prolonged anaesthesia.

Brachial plexus block

This is less easy and best left to the professionals. It can be complicated by a subclavian haematoma or traumatic pneumothorax.

Axillary block

Safer than brachial plexus block, but time-consuming and not always successful.

Femoral nerve block

Should be done on reception of every patient with a fractured shaft of femur; it gives rapid pain-relief and allows skin-traction splintage with comfort and ease. Stand on the contralateral side facing the patient's head; put, and keep, the non-dominant index finger on the femoral artery where it crosses the pelvic brim; inject 10 ml of 0.5% bupivacaine with adrenaline 1/200 000, fan-wise and laterally to the fixed index. Wait 10 minutes and proceed with your manipulations gently, firmly, and swiftly.

Bier's block (intravenous regional block)

This is a very useful technique to produce anaesthesia for the reduction of Colles' fracture and for certain minor surgery on the forearm, wrist, or hand. It is reliable and safe if performed correctly and if a proper cuff (*not a sphygmomanometer cuff*) is used. Proceed as follows:

1 Introduce an in-dwelling needle into a vein in the uninjured arm, to provide rapid access to the circulation in the unlikely event of this being required.
2 Wrap a layer of surgical wool around the upper arm and place the cuff over it. Secure the cuff in place.
3 Position an in-dwelling needle into a vein on the dorsum of the hand on the injured side.
4 Elevate the injured arm for one minute, to collapse the veins.

5   Pump up the cuff to about 250 mm Hg, well above the patient's systolic pressure. Lower the arm.

6   Inject 0.5% prilocaine (40 ml is the usual dose for an adult male).

7   Within 10 minutes, the arm is anaesthetized and surgery can begin.

8   The cuff should not remain inflated for less than 30 minutes or more than 60 minutes.

Intradermal local anaesthesia

See **Abscesses**

Subcutaneous anaesthesia

This is routinely used for minor operations and skin suturing. Do not proceed until you have verified the procedure's effectiveness by testing for absence of pin-prick sensation.

Most of these techniques are well illustrated in Bache *et al. A colour atlas of nursing procedures in accidents and emergencies*: see **Bibliography**.

■ Anaphylaxis, acute

Strictly a hypersensitivity reaction to foreign protein, characterized by an initial sensitizing dose and an out-pouring of histamine or histamine-like substances in response to a second effective dose of the original specific allergen. It can be tissue-specific (e.g. dermal in acute allergic urticaria) or general (e.g. loss of consciousness, asthma, urticaria, cardiac arrhythmia, and peripheral vascular collapse following a wasp sting in a sensitized subject). The term is also loosely used to describe anaphylactoid response to single-dose assaults from such dramatic histaminagogues as snake or scorpion bites, jellyfish and insect stings.

Hypersensitive subjects who may need instant treatment for life-threatening reactions out of range of

immediate medical care should always carry an adrenaline aerosol (e.g. Medihaler-epi), which can be life-saving.

In A & E units the aerosol can be used as a first-aid measure but should be followed by adrenaline 0.1%, 0.5–1 ml intramuscularly, repeated every 15 minutes as required. Intravenous hydrocortisone 100 mg or dexamethasone 5 mg should follow. Severe cases should then be admitted in case of relapse and given chlorpheniramine 10–20 mg slowly intravenously. Milder cases can be discharged on a 5-day course of antihistamines.

Intramuscular adrenaline should be given with great care as it is poorly absorbed in the collapsed patient, but as he recovers a minor overdose given in a moment of panic could be disastrous, especially in a hypertensive subject.

The need for subsequent desensitization must always be remembered and met.

Cf. **Stings, etc. by marine creatures** and **Stings, wasp and bee**

■ Aneurysm, aortic

1 **Arch**—ascending, traditionally (but not reliably) syphilitic; descending, atherosclerotic; may rupture or dissect. The latter is associated with agonizing dorsal pain and interference with peripheral pulses according to the anatomical situation. Rupture kills in a few minutes.

2 **Abdominal** (a) *upper*—severe lumbar pain and shock; (b) *lower*—poorly localized but severe pain in the pelvis, with shock and often interference with the peripheral pulses; may be symmetrical. Early recognition is important now that surgical repair is widely available and skilfully performed by many general surgeons. This can present with testicular pain of great severity.

■ Ankle

Ankle sprains originate in four ways: inversion, over-extension, overflexion, and eversion. Take an accurate history.

Palpate the ankle carefully to determine whether tenderness is maximal over bone or ligament. Palpate the styloid process of the fifth metatarsal at the same time, as avulsion fractures here are common and can be confusing.

X-ray the ankle if there is bony tenderness, or severe pain, or severe swelling, or if the patient is unable to put any weight on the foot, or is elderly, or if the injury fails to settle as quickly as expected, or if the patient/relatives insist that an X-ray is necessary (remember Sod's law!). It has been suggested that a policy of requesting X-ray examination of only those patients with inversion ankle injuries who have distal fibular tenderness or inability to bear weight or are aged over 60, with a further proviso that no foot radiographs should be obtained, would produce a 60% reduction in ankle radiography without detriment to patient care (Dunlop, M. G., Beattie, T. F., White, G. K., Raab, G. M., and Doull, R. I. (1986). Guidelines for selective radiological assessment of inversion ankle injuries. *British Medical Journal*, **293**, 603–5).

Inversion injuries

Commonly the lateral collateral ligaments are strained, or the subtalar joint sprained, or the antero-inferior tibio-fibular ligaments over-stressed. These injuries require only bandage support and active and energetic mobilization. The patient should be told to walk without a limp. It is better not to apply Elastoplast to start with in case of swelling or the need for subsequent X-ray. If pain or disability persist after the fourth day, continue double elastic support, e.g. Tubigrip, for 10–21 days. Ultrasound is helpful if used from the beginning. It relieves pain, reduces swelling, and permits proper movement, which is itself curative.

Some sprains represent partial rupture of the evertor mechanism, i.e. peroneal sprain. These are commonly

associated with extensive bruising above and below the ankle and resolve slowly. Use supporting bandage (see **Bandages**).

Overextension

Can rupture both collateral ligaments and may be associated with compression fracture of the navicular. If it is combined with an axial force (e.g. in jumping from a height) talar fractures can occur and may well need internal fixation.

Overflexion

Can be associated with 'third malleolus' fracture. Look for this on the X-ray. Otherwise anterior capsular injury predominates and may be associated with unimportant flake-fractures from the neck of the talus.

Ruptured ligaments of the ankle

Rupture of ankle ligaments leads to instability of the joint. It is clinically indicated by severe pain and swelling and failure to respond to simple conservative treatment.

Rupture of the medial ligament is demonstrated by stressed eversion radiography (under general anaesthetic). Opinions about treatment differ widely.

Rupture of the lateral ligament may be treated by plaster of Paris for 6 weeks, or by surgical repair. It is demonstrated by stressed inversion radiography (under general anaesthetic).

Rupture of the inferior tibio-fibular ligament (tibio-fibular diastasis) is readily shown by either stressed view, but is relatively rare. It generally requires internal fixation. Sometimes the interosseous ligament may be split as well; the fibular fracture may then be proximal (Maisonneuve injury).

A medial malleolar fracture can be stable (if the periosteum, and thus the medial collateral ligament, is intact) or unstable.

Antibiotics

Partial rupture of the lateral ligamentous/capsular complex shows less marked talar tilt and heals more rapidly than complete rupture. A shorter period (three weeks) in plaster of Paris is needed.

It is high time the best treatment for these conditions was sorted out by adequate controlled trials: they are common enough yet orthopaedic opinion is as variable as April weather. Whatever treatment is required, however, it is essential that the patient elevates his ankle above the level of the waist whenever he is sitting or lying, particularly during the first few days after injury; if he fails to do so, any treatment will give less than satisfactory results.

■ Antibiotics

These should be used as a matter of routine in the following cases:

- Major injuries with soft tissue damage
- All compound fractures
- Head injuries with leakage of cerebrospinal fluid
- Local sepsis which is not subsiding
- Penetrating wounds of hand or foot
- Bites from humans and other animals
- Together with surgery when abscesses are opened (cf. **Abscesses**)
- All tendon injuries
- Crushing injuries of extremities
- Prophylaxis of infection in potentially infected wounds, e.g. hand wounds in meat and poultry handlers
- In all drug addicts requiring anaesthesia for surgical procedures

They should not be used in the following cases:

- Undiagnosed medical infections in children
- Upper respiratory infections of viral origin
- Minor superficial sepsis (impetigo, if severe, can be an exception)
- Uncomplicated skin wounds

It is sometimes difficult to decide which type of antibiotic to use, and the list below may give useful guidance. It is important to remember that a majority of staphylococcal infections is penicillin-resistant (84% in Hereford in 1983) and that a considerable proportion of streptococcal infections is tetracycline-resistant. Therefore:

1 In prophylaxis of infection in wounds and injuries give intramuscular Triplopen (benethamine penicillin 475 mg + procaine penicillin 250 mg + sodium penicillin 300 mg), one vial. If the wound is soiled, or prolonged prophylaxis is desirable, continue with oral Augmentin (= amoxycillin 250 mg + clavulanic acid 125 mg), which is effective against resistant staphylococci, and has an excellent spectrum of activity; dosage suggested for prophylaxis: one Augmentin tablet 8-hourly for 5 days.

2 In obviously staphylococcal infections (localized abscesses, whitlows, etc.) give flucloxacillin 250 mg 4 times a day before food. An increasing number of hand infections show anaerobes on culture. Clindamycin may be considered the antibiotic of first choice, especially if the pus is evil-smelling.

3 In all cases of cellulitis (always streptococcal until proved otherwise) give intramuscular benzylpenicillin 600 mg, followed by oral phenoxymethylpenicillin (Penicillin V) 250 mg 4 times a day before food.

4 In cases of perianal or pararectal abscesses use clindamycin. See **Abscesses**.

5 In cases of penicillin sensitivity which would otherwise call for this class of antibiotic give erythromycin 250–500 mg 4 times a day after food by mouth for 5 days. Clindamycin is sometimes kept in reserve; some recommend it for all penicillin-sensitive patients (cf. **Abscesses**).

6 In cases of head injury where prophylaxis is called for because of suspicion or certainty of meningeal discontinuity, give benzylpenicillin 600 mg, flucloxacillin 500 mg, and sulphadimidine 2 g, all intramuscularly.

7 It is worth recording the high effectiveness of metronidazole in anaerobic infections, particularly those due to *Bacteroides fragilis* (abscesses) and the combination of Vincent's spirochaetes and fusiforms which are the causative organisms of acute ulcerative gingivo-stomatitis. Recent advances in the management of abscesses and hand infections highlight the frequency of anaerobic infections. In general clindamycin is the best drug for these. Cf. **Abscesses.**

8 Clearly, subsequent bacteriological findings may modify these guidelines, but you must start somewhere.

The use of a single dose of antibiotic at the time of injury is intended to prevent the multiplication of externally-entering contaminants. Practice suggests that it is effective provided the spectrum of cover is wide and the dose adequate. It is not likely to encourage the development of resistant strains as longer courses certainly will. This point of view has become increasingly acceptable in traditional surgical circles in the last few years. Recently published work extends the application to abscesses. Cf. **Abscesses.**

In using antibiotics the worst single crime you can commit is to use them ineffectively, i.e. in inadequate dosage or of irrelevant spectrum.

Penicillin sensitivity

Many patients claim allergy to penicillin. Often they refer to minor gastrointestinal disturbances on taking an antibiotic many years ago. Take a careful history and do not give penicillins or cephalosporins if allergy seems genuine (e.g. urticaria or angio-oedema). There is no convenient and absolutely reliable method of identifying patients at risk of developing reactions to penicillin (Beeley, L. (1984). Allergy to penicillin. *British Medical Journal* **288**, 511–12). If in doubt, use an alternative antibiotic.

Antiseptics

Tincture of iodine should be used generally for epidermal injuries, especially if caused by cats, rabbits, rats or other rodents, mad dogs, or humans. Rabid dog bites should be treated with copious applications of tincture of iodine as soon as possible. Cf. **Bites**, **Rabies**.

Other topical antiseptics include:

- Chlorhexidine
- Eusol (Edinburgh University Solution of Lime)
- Hydrogen peroxide solution
- Proflavine cream
- Silver sulphadiazine cream
- Povidone-iodine ointment

Their uses are illustrated in Bache *et al. A colour atlas of nursing procedures in accidents and emergencies*: see **Bibliography**.

Artefact injuries

Must not be forgotten in diagnosis. Differential diagnosis is established by making the lesion inaccessible by appropriate bandaging or plaster of Paris. Unravelling the underlying psychogenic factors is no part of the casualty officer's job.

If a presenting condition does not make sense (e.g. an apyrexial patient with a red, hot swelling but a normal white cell count), suspect artefact.

■ Asphyxia

The numerous causes include:

- Laryngeal occlusion by food (see **Foreign bodies**)
- Laryngeal occlusion by swelling, secretions, or vomiting in the unconscious (see **Head injuries**)
- Severe acute asthma (q.v.)
- Drowning (q.v.) (water, blood, or vomit can drown)
- Facial injuries (see **Fractures, maxillo-facial injuries**)
- Acute pulmonary oedema (see **Asthma, cardiac**)
- Chest injuries (q.v.)
- Anaphylaxis (q.v.) (e.g. wasp-sting sensitivity) (see **Stings, wasp and bee**)
- Angio-oedema (cf. **Anaphylaxis, acute**)
- Epiglottitis (see **Stridor, acute**)
- Laryngeal oedema (croup, etc.)

■ Assault, physical

Serious assaults often lead to multiple injuries and the victim is often drunk, or a bad witness, or both. If in doubt, admit. Injuries from assault are a growing epidemic in Britain.

■ Assault, sexual

A police surgeon, not a casualty officer, should examine such a case.

If circumstances compel you to perform this duty, the patient must be stripped completely and notes taken carefully of every injury and mark on the skin. Nails are particularly important: scrapings from under a girl's nails may give vital evidence. Note general appearance, clothing, stains, soiling of garments, emotional state. Take the following specimens to examine for spermatozoa:

- Moist swab from perineum
- Moist swab from vulva
- Moist swab from vagina
- Moist swab from pubic hair
- Clippings of pubic hair, into a sterile bottle

Give all specimens to the police for examination at a forensic laboratory.

Always have a chaperon/witness.

Be prepared to be humiliated mercilessly and publicly in court by learned counsel.

■ Asthma, bronchial

Essentially a complaint for management and supervision by the General Practitioner; but from time to time severe attacks of breathlessness reach A & E departments. Severity is indicated by cyanosis, tachycardia, inability to speak due to dyspnoea, or a 'silent chest'. The peak expiratory flow rate should be measured on arrival and arterial blood gases should be measured as soon as possible. A chest X-ray should be performed at an early stage, to eliminate the possibility of a pneumothorax. Treatment is as follows:

1 **Salbutamol nebulization** 0.5 ml of respirator solution (5 mg/ml) in 2 ml of normal saline for children under 12 years; 1 ml of respirator solution in 4 ml of saline for adults. Salbutamol is a selective β_2-adreno-ceptor stimulant. This is outstandingly the best emergency treatment. The solution is put into the receptacle of the nebulizer attached to a standard oxygen mask and nebulized by the hospital **oxygen** supply. Its action is gentle, rapid, and efficient. The rate and quantity of the nebulization is determined by its effects. Nebulization can also be done by electrically driven air-pump, or by air compressed by foot-pump: various models are available. **Terbutaline** is an alternative to salbutamol, and can also be given by nebulization.

2 **Aminophylline** (a xanthine bronchodilator) by intravenous injection, 250–500 mg (5 mg/kg for children) given slowly over 20 minutes and followed by a continuous infusion at a rate of 1 mg/kg/h. Plasma concentrations should be monitored prior to treatment, particularly if patients have been taking oral xanthine preparations, as serious side-effects, such as convulsions and arrhythmias, can occasionally occur before the appearance of other symptoms of toxicity; if concentrations are unavailable, omit the loading dose of aminophylline prior to the infusion.

3 **Steroids** have an important adjuvant role in acute, severe asthma. They are secondary to the above remedies as they are slow-acting. Hydrocortisone sodium succinate 200 mg intravenously is appropriate: its onset time is 2–4 hours.

4 **Sedation** should be avoided but massive reassurance works wonders.

5 **Intravenous fluids** should be started early in severe cases, especially children, to avoid dehydration.

Any patient, child or adult, who has required nebulization or intravenous therapy should be admitted, or at least be assessed by a paediatrician or physician.

■ Asthma, cardiac

An acute pulmonary oedema due to left-sided heart failure. Treat as follows:

- **Sit the patient up**.
- Give **oxygen**: if there is definitely no past history of lung disease, give 100% oxygen and sedate the patient with **diamorphine** 5 mg intravenously; if the patient has a history of previous lung disease, give 24% oxygen.
- Give an intravenous **diuretic** (e.g. frusemide 80 mg) and repeat if necessary.
- **Aminophylline**, 250 mg slowly intravenously, can be given if the patient is in sinus rhythm.
- If the patient isn't on digoxin already, digitalization may be needed too, especially if the patient is in fast atrial fibrillation: intravenous **digoxin** 0.5 mg, repeated if necessary.

Early investigations include a chest X-ray, an ECG (has the patient had a myocardial infarct?), urea and electrolytes, cardiac enzymes, haemoglobin and full blood count, and arterial blood gases.

■ Backs

Half the population suffers from backache, owing to misuse or disuse (the latter more prevalent). The other half is still liable to back injury or disease. The commonest manifestations are:

1 **Acute lumbago**. See **Lumbago**.

2 **Chronic backache** may well need investigation of lumbar spine and sacro-iliac joints, gynaecological apparatus, and psychosexual background. Treatment: once organic disease is excluded, vigorous mobilization and extension exercises. A day's digging or some all-in wrestling is excellent. Manipulation is good in experienced hands. This is not strictly an emergency commitment however.

3   **Prolapsed intervertebral disc** should not be diagnosed without symptoms or signs of root-pressure, e.g. limitation of straight-leg raising or other root pain. The severe, acute prolapsed intervertebral disc is usually well dealt with by means of a plaster of Paris jacket — three weeks in the first instance. The patient should be warned that it may be 10 days before the root pain subsides. If the pain is intolerable, admission for rest and traction is occasionally required. See **Neuropathies**.

4   **Ligamentous injury**, especially interspinous ligament injury: local tenderness is acute. Inject bupivacaine 0.5%, 5 ml at least, and mobilize.

5   **Quadratus lumborum myalgia** (with or without exertion fracture of the twelfth rib). Infiltrate with local bupivacaine 0.5% 10 ml, and mobilize. Avoid renal biopsy.

6   **Dorsago** is an acute dorsal syndrome involving the erector spinae or serratus posterior, comparable in its characteristics to acute lumbago; it is common and can be very painful and disabling. Infiltration of local anaesthetic around the relevant costo-vertebral or interfacetal joint can be dramatically helpful. Painful muscle spasms are particularly distressing. If precise localization is impossible inject three or four boluses of 5 ml bupivacaine 0.25% deep into the paravertebral muscles; this will generally control the painful spasms.

Back injuries are dealt with under **Fractures, spine**.

Pathological fractures, Pott's disease, and other medical mysteries should always be borne in mind but are not strictly an A & E commitment.

Physiotherapists have much to offer to acute cases of lumbago and to the re-education of the backs of recurrent sufferers. See **Physiotherapy**.

■ Bandages

Supporting bandages

It is frequently desirable to use supporting bandages for the following purposes:

- Control of oedema
- Support of injured bones and joints
- Improvement of blood supply in the lower limb

The available types of support include:

- Elasticated tubular support (Tubigrip)
- Crêpe bandage
- Elastic adhesive tape (Elastoplast)

Crêpe bandage is useful for only 4 hours and then needs expert reapplication. Elastoplast is good but tiresome to remove, and often produces skin reactions; it is also partially radio-opaque. Tubigrip is as good as any and has no disadvantages; all patients should be told to remove it at night if it is uncomfortable, and reapply it before rising. Don't forget that *all wounds of the leg and foot require toe-to-knee support.*

Ichthopaste bandages

Ichthopaste (zinc oxide 6% and ichthammol 2% paste impregnated on bandage) is a very useful and comfortable application for wounds and skin lesions in atrophic skins, or in the presence of poor blood supply in the leg. It should always be applied from the toes to the knee. It can often be left in place for one or two weeks at a time. Ichthopaste can often be used where there is infection or an eczematous skin, in combination with topical anti-septics and saline bathing. It is softer and more comfort-able than plain zinc-paste bandages, besides containing ichthammol as a stimulant to epidermal growth; it is a very useful dressing for slow healing hand and finger wounds, especially where the volar skin is hard and thick.

■ Bites

Dog

Bruising is often more significant than laceration. Tetanus immunization is essential. Give intramuscular Triplopen, followed by oral Augmentin if the wound is soiled (see **Antibiotics**). Dress the wound with tincture of iodine. The common dog-bites of the face in children need early and careful repair (often under general anaesthesia). *Pasteurella septica/multocida* is an important pathogen from dog and cat bites and is sensitive to Augmentin. Cf. **Rabies**.

Cat

Needs to be treated with extra respect because of the risk of cat-bite/scratch fever. Dress with tincture of iodine and give intramuscular Triplopen as above. Again remember tetanus immunization.

Pig

Pigs have very strong jaws and can inflict a lot of tissue damage and/or fractures through undamaged skin and clothing. Treat all symptoms with respect.

Horse

Usually a superficial nip. A case where a jealous stallion grabbed his handler by the scrotum, picked him up and shook him, then dropped him on his back, was exciting but unusual. *Actinobacillus lignieresii* from horses and cattle can infect man and a bacteriologist should be consulted.

Snake

The adder is the only poisonous snake native to Britain. Bites generally produce local symptoms only, and disproportionate fear. Snake-bite serum should not be used automatically. Admit for observation. Treatment is symptomatic and, in the rare cases of general poisoning with collapse (histamine-type symptoms), intravenous fluids and general supportive treatment are necessary. See **Poisoning**. To patients genuinely collapsed at first contact give intramuscular adrenaline (0.5 ml of 0.1%, repeated every 15 minutes as required) and intravenous hydrocortisone 100 mg or dexamethasone 4 mg. The main indication for antivenom therapy is systemic envenoming.

Detailed advice on the management of bites by poisonous snakes is available from the Liverpool School of Tropical Medicine (051-708-9393), or the Radcliffe Infirmary, Oxford (0865-249891), or the National Poisons Information Centre (01-407-7600).

See H. A. Reid's chapter 'Poisoning due to snake bite' in Vale and Meredith, *Poisoning: diagnosis and treatment* (see **Bibliography**).

Insect

Even the angriest looking swelling is generally an alkaloid reaction or an allergic one. Secondary infection is rare and generally accompanied by lymphangitis. Therefore an antihistamine is the first treatment to try. See **Stings, wasp and bee**.

Spider

A useful review article (Anonymous (1980). Spider bites. *Lancet*, **ii**, 133-4) largely exonerates *Lycosa tarantula* from seriously morbid effects and directs attention to *Latrodectus tredecimguttatus*. The female of the latter species is black or brown with usually 13 (as its name implies) red spots; its bite is said to give 5% mortality. Muscular cramps and hypertension are characteristic and a specific antivenom is available. Otherwise treatment is supportive.

Man

Often met with after fights; aimed at inflicting maximum damage to ears, noses, fingers, etc. Treat on general lines. Human bites must never be considered trivial (Kirkpatrick, B. and Wise, R. (1986). *British Medical Journal*, **293**, 1522–3).

■ Blisters

Whether due to burning, friction, or unknown causes, blisters provide a good sterile dressing, and are best left for a few days. If they burst or merely persist after five days they should never be pricked, but removed in their entirety. Appropriate treatment can then be given to the deeper tissues disclosed by their removal. Pricking can only introduce infection into a sterile medium ideally suited to the multiplication of bacteria.

Cold epidermolysis often puzzles people. It presents as a brownish blister of the sole in cold or damp winter weather. Sometimes this becomes painful. If recurrent, early injection of intralesional methylprednisolone (Depo-Medrone) will abort it.

■ Burns

Severe burns

For a severely burnt patient (over 10% surface area in a child; over 15% in an adult), proceed as follows:

1   Ensure there is a satisfactory airway. Give oxygen. Give nebulized salbutamol if necessary (see **Asthma, bronchial**).
2   Set up an intravenous infusion, using as large a cannula as possible. Use saline initially, then Haemaccel as soon as you are satisfied with the vein; go on to plasma protein fraction when it is available.

3 Give analgesia: intravenous morphine (0.1–0.2 mg/kg) is best.

4 Take blood for haemoglobin, full blood count, packed cell volume, urea and electrolytes, arterial blood gases, carboxyhaemoglobin level, and group and save serum. Record the pulse and blood pressure.

5 Cover the burnt areas with sterile towels, soaked in saline.

6 Inform the general surgeons or the plastic surgeons.

7 Estimate the volume of intravenous fluid which is required. To do this you will need to know (a) the time of the accident; (b) the percentage surface area burnt (don't include simple erythema; see Figs 2 and 3); (c) the weight of the patient. Various formulae are used to calculate this. The simplest is:

A = volume of fluid required over the first 4 hours after burning

= (% area burnt × weight of patient (kg) × $\frac{1}{2}$) ml

This same volume will be required over hours 4–8, 8–12, 12–18, 18–24, and 24–36; however, re-assessment will be needed at frequent intervals, taking into account clinical state, urine output, packed cell volume, etc. Give equal amounts of saline and colloid (Haemaccel or plasma protein fraction) in A & E. Whole blood may be needed later if there has been much full thickness burning. Sodium bicarbonate may be needed to correct acidosis.

8 Give tetanus prophylaxis if required.

9 Catheterize the bladder and start a fluid balance chart.

By this stage, the patient should have been transferred to the appropriate surgeons.

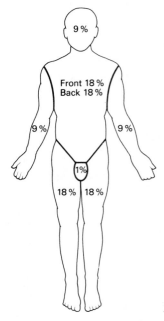

Fig. 2. Simple 'rule of nines' for rapid estimation of total body area burnt in adults.

Reasons for admission include:

- Large burns needing intravenous therapy
- Inhalation of smoke or steam: airway involvement
- Particular nursing problems: hands, eyes, face, perineum, circumferential burns of limbs or chest or neck (may need escharotomy), very young or very old patients
- Possible non-accidental injury in children
- Full thickness burns for early surgery

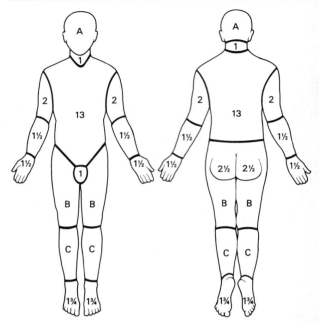

Fig. 3. Estimation of percentage of total body area burnt in children by Lund and Browder charts.

Smaller burns

Most departments have a burns clinic in one form or another, to deal with those patients who do not require specialist treatment as in-patients. Such clinics have two great advantages:

1 It is possible to arrange for the same person to see the patient on each visit. It is very difficult to determine whether or not a burn is improving if you are seeing it for the first time.

2 Experience is invaluable in the treatment of burns. It is extremely difficult to describe when to change from one type of dressing to another; often it is no more than a gut feeling. One or two nurses in a unit

Relative percentage of areas affected by growth

Age in years	0	1	5	10	15	Adult
A — ½ of head	9½	8½	6½	5½	4½	3½
B — ½ of one thigh	2¾	3¼	4	4¼	4½	4¾
C — ½ of one leg	2½	2½	2¾	3	3¼	3½

tend to take a particular interest in burns and develop great experience over the years; cultivate them and learn from them: no book can replace them.

Full thickness burns (detected by loss of sensation to pin prick) may well require grafting, unless the full thickness area is small, in which case normal skin will slowly advance from the edges. However, scar tissue results in contractures, which are unsightly and restrict movement.

If you feel that skin grafting may be necessary, bring the patient to the attention of your consultant, so that he can arrange grafting at an early stage; a 10-day delay may reveal the fact that a burn which was initially thought to be full thickness is, in fact, partly or entirely partial thickness.

So far as dressings are concerned, debris is removed and I then tend to apply 1% silver sulphadiazine (Flamazine) cream and cover this with a non-adherent dressing. Dressings are usually needed thrice weekly initially. Once the burn is under control (i.e. not becoming infected and obviously mostly partial thickness), I dress the area with povidone iodine non-adherent dressing (Inadine) to dry it and continue using this until it can be left open. Lanolin and salt baths may be useful at this stage to prevent the skin from drying and cracking.

Different units have different preferences: become acquainted with yours.

Particular problems

Burns to the face Oxytetracycline and hydrocortisone (Terra-Cortril) spray is excellent. Exclude inhalation burns, which cause increasingly severe symptoms over 48 hours.

Burns to the eyelids Ensure the eyes themselves are undamaged; seek ophthalmological help if necessary.

Burns to the hand Early mobilization is essential to prevent severe stiffness. Spread 1% silver sulphadiazine (Flamazine) cream over the area of the burn and cover the hand with a burn bag, anchored around the wrist. Stress

the necessity of elevation and mobilization. Daily dressings will be needed. This treatment is very messy and quite uncomfortable and the patient becomes worried by the macerated skin but it is beautifully effective in overcoming the problem of stiffness. Early physiotherapy is invaluable.

Burns to the limbs   A circumferential burn to a limb may need escharotomy to prevent ischaemia: the dead skin is divided longitudinally from one end of the burn to the other (Brown, J. and Ward, D. J. (1984). Immediate management of burns in casualty. *British Journal of Hospital Medicine*, **31**, 360–8); this is painless if the burn is full thickness.

Non-accidental burns in children   These include cigarette burns, burns with hot irons, burns of the perineum, or glove or stocking burns from dipping a hand or foot in hot water. See **Child abuse**.

Hydrofluoric acid burns   After copious irrigation with water, apply 2.5% calcium gluconate gel to the skin or 10% calcium gluconate solution to the eyes.

Chemical burns   Irrigate liberally with cold water, but avoid hypothermia!

Bitumen burns   Cool with water and remove the bitumen by very gentle washing with diesel oil; forcible removal is unnecessary as any remaining bitumen will gradually separate. If the hands are involved, complete removal is important, so that early mobilization is possible.

Electrical burns   These may well be full thickness and the area of necrosis may extend over the first few days. Consult a plastic surgeon on the day of injury, as he may wish to excise and graft then. The current may flow along structures such as nerves or vessels.

Cf. **Adhesives**

Burns: the first 48 hours by J. A. D. Settle is available from Smith and Nephew Pharmaceuticals Ltd., Bampton Road, Harold Hill, Romford, Essex RM3 8SL. It is well worth reading. Obtain a copy for yourself and ensure one is available in your unit.

■ Bursitis

The treatment for this condition is *rest* and protection. In acute olecranon or pre-patellar bursitis, even when grossly inflamed, the fluid contents are generally sterile. *Primary aspiration is absolutely contra-indicated in all severe cases.* It all too often results in either infection or a chronic sinus or both. In the subacute or chronic phase aspiration and introduction of methylprednisolone (Depo-Medrone) is helpful, and may materially shorten the disability and pain. Puncture should be made at the least dependent point. Full sterile precautions in theatre should be observed. A purulent bursitis is a rarity and generally the outcome of meddlesome treatment. If it occurs it is still best treated conservatively with anti-biotics and rest.

Pre-patellar bursitis settles rapidly in a well-padded plaster cylinder.

Recurrent bursitis should be referred, failing all else, to the General Practitioner for formal surgical removal of the bursa to be arranged, or directly to an orthopaedic surgeon if you are permitted to do this. Don't excise bursae yourself as healing over bony prominences (e.g. the olecranon) is often very unsatisfactory. Leave this to a specialist.

■ Cardiac arrest

There is much controversy regarding the finer details of management, and the standards of resuscitation perform-ance among the junior medical staff in Britain leave a lot of room for improvement (Baskett, P. J. F. (1985). Resuscitation needed for the curriculum? *British Medical Journal*, **290**, 1531–2). The Resuscitation Council (UK) has drawn up guidelines for both basic and advanced life support and these are available from the Department of Anaesthetics, Royal Postgraduate Medical School, Du Cane Road, London W12 0HS. The poster 'Cardio-pulmonary Resuscitation' should be prominently dis-played in the resuscitation room and elsewhere. Clever

medical registrars, bristling with inexperience, may disagree with the details but their wiser colleagues recognize its value.

It is imperative that you know how to use all the equipment *before* the necessity arises.

1   Establish a diagnosis: the patient is unconscious with absent pulse and/or respiration.

2   Call for help. Summon the cardiac arrest team.

3   Ensure the airway is clear (remove dentures, secretions, vomit, etc.; extend the neck and lift the chin forwards; insert a Guedel airway). Get air into the lungs either by mouth-to-mouth respiration or with a bag and mask. Begin external cardiac massage. If you are still alone, do 15 chest compressions to 2 inflations.
A = airway
B = breathing
C = circulation

4   When help arrives, connect the patient to an ECG monitor to establish the rhythm of the heart: the details of further management depend upon this. There are three likely rhythms: ventricular fibrillation, asystole, and electromechanical dissociation (the ECG shows QRS complexes but there is no heart beat). If the tracing is flat, check the connections, switches and gain.

5   Ensure that the patient is now getting oxygen, rather than air. Endotracheal intubation should be established as soon as a competent intubator is available (Scott, D. B. (1986). Endotracheal intubation: friend or foe. *British Medical Journal*, **292**, 157–8). Cannulate a large vein (e.g. the external jugular).

6   **Ventricular fibrillation (VF)**
(a) Charge up the defibrillator to 200 J and give this shock to the patient (one paddle is at the apex and the other is below the right clavicle; ensure there is a good electrical contact by using conducting gel pads; ensure no one is touching the patient or the trolley when the shock is given—even medical students mustn't be exterminated like that!).

(b) If VF continues, give a second 200 J shock.

(c) If that fails, give a 400 J shock.

(d) If VF remains, give lignocaine 100 mg intravenously (or 200 mg endotracheally).

(e) Next try another 400 J shock.

(f) If unsuccessful, give adrenaline 10 ml of 0.01% intravenously (or 20 ml of 0.01% endotracheally).

(g) Try another 400 J shock.

(h) Give 50 ml of 8.4% sodium bicarbonate intravenously at this stage if you've still had no success.

(i) Then try another 400 J shock.

(j) If the VF persists to this stage, you can try further lignocaine or bretylium tosylate 500 mg intravenously or other anti-arrhythmics before giving further 400 J shocks. An intravenous infusion of lignocaine (3 mg/min) may help.

NB Interruption of basic life support (ventilations and compressions) must be minimal as these sequences are followed, until an effective heart beat is re-established; the ECG takes 5–10 seconds to recover after defibrillation and cannot be interpreted during this time. Therefore check a major pulse within three seconds of defibrillation and, if there is no pulse, administer 15 more chest compressions and then read the ECG.

7 **Asystole**

(a) Give atropine 1 mg intravenously (or 2 mg endotracheally).

(b) If asystole persists, give adrenaline 10 ml of 0.01% intravenously (or 20 ml of 0.01% endotracheally).

(c) If unsuccessful, give 50 ml of 8.4% sodium bicarbonate intravenously.

(d) Next try isoprenaline 100 μg intravenously.

(e) If asystole persists to this stage, you can try intracardiac adrenaline (10 ml of 0.01%). Pacing may help if there is any evidence of electrical activity.

8 **Electromechanical dissociation**

(a) Consider the possibility of drugs, cardiac tamponade (q.v.), tension pneumothorax (q.v.) exsanguination, or other physical causes. Treat these appropriately.

(b) Give adrenaline 10 ml of 0.01% intravenously (or 20 ml of 0.01% endotracheally).

(c) If no success, give isoprenaline 100 μg intravenously.

(d) Consider giving calcium chloride 10 ml of 10% intravenously.

During or immediately after resuscitation, check the patient's urea and electrolytes, arterial blood gases, and get a chest X-ray.

(The above doses are those for a 70 kg male.)

Between April and July 1986, the *British Medical Journal* published an excellent series of articles under the heading of 'ABC of resuscitation'. These were followed by a considerable volume of correspondence. These articles are now available as a book, edited by T. R. Evans: see **Bibliography**.

■ Cardiac failure, acute congestive

See **Asthma, cardiac**

■ Cardiac tamponade

Difficult to diagnose and often missed, with fatal results. If it is spotted it may be curable. It can be due to crush injury leading to bursting of the myocardium, or penetrating wounds from external (metallic fragments) or internal (rib penetration) causes. Not an uncommon steering-wheel injury in car accidents.

'Medical' haemato-pericardium due to the ruptured scar of a previous infarction, or to a dissecting aneurysm of the ascending aorta, is for practical purposes a terminal event.

Clinical diagnosis   Accelerating pulse and falling blood pressure in the absence of evident blood loss. Rapid rise of jugular venous pressure. Sudden cardiac arrest ensues and is usually irreversible.

Confirmatory diagnosis   Pericardial paracentesis using a wide-bore needle into the angle between the seventh left costal cartilage and the xiphisternum, directing the needle upwards and backwards.

Treatment   Urgent surgical repair.

■ Cardiovascular emergencies, other

Cardiovascular collapse can also be caused (especially in elderly people with poor cardiac reserves) by dissecting *aneurysm* of the aorta or major peripheral *embolism*. Now that vascular surgery is widely available, early diagnosis and referral are urgent. The collapsed patient with absent femoral pulses may have a saddle embolus at the bifurcation or a low dissection of the aortic wall. Femoral embolism, or even popliteal, can present with collapse as well as signs of arterial occlusion, and both may be amenable to urgent surgery.

Heart block is readily diagnosed clinically and by ECG but intermittent heart block with occasional Stokes–Adams syncopal attacks may be undetectable except by 24-hour ECG.

Rare causes include visceral embolism (especially mesenteric), intermittent mitral obstruction (due to intra-atrial thrombosis or pedunculated myxoma), acute toxic myocarditis (e.g. after influenza), and, among those suffering from starvation, beri-beri heart.

Pulmonary embolism should always be borne in mind, even in the absence of evidence of previous deep venous thrombosis.

Cf. **Myocardial infarction** and **Collapse and coma**

■ Caustics

Strong acids make painful burns on the skin and so generally get rapid treatment. Strong alkalis and phenols, unfortunately, are generally painless and may not be recognized as caustic. As a result their caustic onset is insidious and more disastrous. Its full extent may not be recognized for several weeks, e.g. on the back of the hand, where primary tendon damage may pass unrecognized. When children drink any of the many caustics in the home (e.g. alkaline domestic cleaners) there is a strong case for considering admission to a chest unit where oesophagoscopy can if necessary be followed by operation to close mediastinal leaks from the oesophagus.

See also **Poisoning**

■ Chest injuries

Fractures of the ribs or costal cartilages are clinical diagnoses: specific tender site(s), acute pain on coughing and laughing and deep inspiration. X-rays are only needed to confirm or eliminate underlying damage to the heart, lungs or diaphragm; oblique views help to show up the fractures but the more anterior they are, the more difficult they are to see on X-rays. Strapping should be avoided as it predisposes to infection. A sling on the relevant side gives comfort, and local bupivacaine 0.5% gives temporary relief: block the intercostal nerves involved at least 10 cm proximal to the fracture site, and the nerves immediately above and below. Pain is severe for 2 weeks but there is considerable discomfort for 10 weeks or so. The elderly and others with poor respiratory reserve before injury are particularly prone to atelectasis and pneumonia; adequate analgesia and physiotherapy are essential.

Penetrating and crushing injuries of the chest are always serious and can be rapidly fatal if not dealt with expeditiously. Perforations or lacerations of the lung can rapidly embarrass respiration by *pneumothorax, haemothorax,*

or considerable swelling. Ask for the patient's consent to test each X-rays if pneumothorax or haemothorax are suspected. If the first radiograph is negative, and should be done at the second on control part of the midclavicular line. The lateral film on each side can be used in an emergency to show that there is a ruptured diaphragm with liver or stomach in the chest. The transparent medial-mediastinal X-rays rather are here to show field for surgical emphysema and look for the X-rays, the draw ruptured diaphragm. If liver or stomach these may otherwise be missed and a chest drain inserted may increase intrathoracic pressure.

Tension pneumothorax is probably the most urgent diagnosis you will ever have to make, and do so without a further X-rays. Decompression and drainage can be life-saving.

X-rays a patient with a tension pneumothorax of a large pneumothorax rapidly becomes respiratory compromised. Clinical signs are hollow, and remember that the pleural space and the superior vena cava shift and the trachea (with the large veins and the heart), the lung is then not compressed, the veins are compressed, and the tissues with the pressure is approximately atmospheric. Unless you think to check for these in a major injury case you will then be dealt with at a post-mortem exam. Make sure you do this and see the same that you see on film.

Flail segment. There is often a relation of paradoxical respiratory movement of the chest wall when the patient coughs, may be seen easily with the patient in supine position. Try to identify the entire segment aged for ambulatory and treatment. Fixation of the flail segment and occasional early surgery resolves the problem by ventilation. Do your best, and remember that the flail segment also implies considerable trauma of the chest wall.

Depressed sternum. Look for associated features, and for pain on movement, and for tenderness over the sternum.

Mediastinal structures. Be aware of the serious injuries to the chest that follow rapid deceleration, and more often is seen here than the physician would expect.

or a combination of both. Ask for inspiration and expiration chest X-rays if pneumothorax or haemothorax are suspected. Early intercostal intubation is safe and should be done in the second intercostal space in the midclavicular line. The lateral approach should never be used in an emergency as there may be a ruptured diaphragm with liver or stomach in the chest. The transparent trochar-mounted (Argyle) tubes are best. Always feel for *surgical emphysema* and look for it on X-rays; it draws attention to injuries of lungs or bronchi which may otherwise be missed. Erect chest radiographs tell much more than supine ones.

Tension pneumothorax is probably the most urgent diagnosis you will ever meet (other than cardiac arrest). Patients die within minutes and there is no time for an X-ray. A patient with the clinical features of a large pneumothorax, rapidly becoming increasingly dyspnoeic, should have a hollow needle inserted into the pleural space on the relevant side; his tension pneumothorax (with its pressure well above atmospheric) is thus converted into a common-or-garden pneumothorax (with its pressure at approximately atmospheric), which can then be dealt with at a slightly more relaxed pace. When you do this, air whooshes out and you save a life.

Flail segment, diagnosed by observation of paradoxical respiration and particularly obvious when the patient coughs, may be extensive and rapidly produce respiratory embarrassment, quickly leading to death, especially in aged or emphysematous patients. Fixation of the flail segment and endotracheal intubation solves the problem by enabling positive pressure ventilation, so that the flail segment once again moves in harmony with the rest of the chest wall.

Depressed sternal fractures are intensely painful. Admit for pain relief and cardiac monitoring in case of arrhythmias.

Mediastinal haemorrhage may follow from compression injuries of the chest, especially in the elderly in whom quite small arteries, brittle from degenerative changes,

may bleed slowly and unnoticed. The signs are of rising pulse rate and falling blood pressure, and rapidly increasing jugular venous filling and jugular venous pulse, in a chest-injured patient who shows no apparent blood loss and normal lung fields. There may be no observable fracture. There is, however, progressive widening of the mediastinal shadow on serial X-rays. The internal mammary artery is usually the culprit.

Adult respiratory distress syndrome (shock lung) is a condition due to major blood loss in which blood volume replacement has been inadequate or delayed. The basic lesion is disseminated intravascular coagulation (DIC). The causative role of surfactant disturbance is not yet clear. There is considerable evidence that large doses of steroids materially reduce the severity of DIC and its consequences. Methylprednisolone sodium succinate (Solu-Medrone) 2 g should be given intravenously at the earliest opportunity if there is any likelihood of its development.

Lung contusion is not necessarily associated with any rib fractures. It may initiate DIC and warrants the same treatment. The clinical condition can deteriorate dramatically over the first 48–72 hours, so that a patient can be sent home on the day of injury and be admitted severely ill a few days later.

Mediastinal compression is recognized by the development of petechial haemorrhages in the skin of the chest and shoulders above the line of compression (e.g. by accidents in civil engineering). Snowstorm petechiae in the lungs also develop and may produce symptoms. The same treatment may be worth using.

Blast-lung (pulmonary barotrauma) is also associated with DIC. Steroids are well worth trying, together with all other supportive care available.

Injuries to the heart and great vessels can be penetrating (urgent thoracotomy can be life-saving) or blunt. The latter can result in tears of the atria or ventricles, cardiac tamponade (q.v.), valvular insufficiency or arrhythmias

Child abuse

(see Bancewicz, J., and Yates, D. (1983). Blunt injury to the heart. *British Medical Journal*, **286**, 497–8). Rupture of the ascending aorta or the arch is almost invariably rapidly fatal.

Injuries to the diaphragm can result from blunt or penetrating trauma and symptoms may be minimal or obscured; careful study of an erect chest X-ray is essential.

Serious chest injuries need early transfer to intensive therapy. Arterial blood gases should be measured soon after arrival. Patients surviving serious chest injuries usually return to their pre-accident state; this is untrue for many other injuries (e.g. head or limbs).

Cf. **Thoracic intubation**

■ Child abuse

Injuries to children are usually quite innocent but factors suggesting that they are non-accidental include the following:

- Delay in presentation
- Apparent lack of concern by the parent(s); contrariwise they may appear over-anxious
- Inadequate or implausible explanation: a baby is most unlikely to break its leg by falling from a settee onto a carpeted floor; 2-month-old infants don't fall out of cots
- Clinical or radiological evidence of multiple injuries, particularly of different ages
- Withdrawn or frightened or very nervous or quiet child

Factors making abuse more likely include:

- Single parent families
- Young parents
- Youngest or unwanted child
- Parental isolation
- Parental alcoholism, drug-taking, or criminal history
- Parental depression or psychiatric history
- Parental stress, including unemployment, financial problems, social problems, or accommodation problems
- Several children in rapid succession or new pregnancy or recent delivery
- Failure to gain weight
- Feeding difficulties
- Frequent medical consultations (at the General Practitioner's or in Accident and Emergency): an 'at-risk' register should be kept; computerized records are of great value in this respect

Teachers may give valuable evidence if the abuse involves children of school age.

Any injury may be non-accidental but be particularly suspicious of possible cigarette burns, scalds, human bites, retinal haemorrhages, skull fractures, rib fractures, metaphysial chip fractures, bruises possibly due to violent grasping or prodding or shaking, and tears of the frenulum. The bones of infants are supple and one child in eight aged under 18 months who sustains a fracture may be a victim of child abuse (see Worlock, P., Stower, M., and Barbor, P. (1986). Patterns of fractures in accidental and non-accidental injury in children: a comparative study. *British Medical Journal*, **293**, 100–2).

Examine the child fully and record your findings accurately with diagrams, which may later be required when giving evidence in court. Photographs should be taken if possible: record when they were taken and by whom.

If you suspect child abuse, handle the situation very delicately and don't mention your suspicions to the parents at this early stage. *Admit the child*. It may be

necessary to persuade the parents, for example by saying that all fractures need admitting to exclude vascular injury, or that it is advisable to admit children with marked bruising to do a platelet count, or children with fractures to exclude osteogenesis imperfecta. But ensure that the admitting team, surgical or orthopaedic, and above all the paediatric team are not deceived regarding the true reason for admission. Discuss the case directly with an experienced paediatrician.

Very rarely, parents refuse admission, probably because they know of your suspicions. If persuasion fails, you can obtain a Place of Safety Order, with the urgent help of a social worker. In any event, inform your consultant and a senior paediatrician at an early stage.

Skeletal surveys should not be requested by a casualty officer; if you are sufficiently worried to think these necessary, then admission is mandatory.

Even more difficult is the problem of sexual abuse of children. The offender is often a member or close acquaintance of the family and it is becoming increasingly common (see Wild, N. J. (1986). Sexual abuse of children in Leeds. *British Medical Journal*, **292**, 1113–16). Again ensure that the child is admitted and the paediatricians are fully aware of the situation. Cf. **Assault, sexual**.

The term child abuse also includes nutritional and emotional deprivation. Parents may fabricate an illness in the child, or withhold medical care.

Overlapping with this problem is that of parental incompetence. It is not your duty to judge, although you are perfectly entitled to your opinion and have a right to express it. Every day, a parent is asked why his child has not been immunized and replies, 'I don't agree with it.' (Response: 'Do you agree with him getting tetanus?') The parents' opinions on such diverse subjects as hygiene, school attendance, dental care, diet, vocabulary, manners, bed-time, playing on busy roads, immunization, smoking, suitable recreation, etc., may well not tally with your own. You would be ill-advised to point out the law of the land, as frequently the parents don't worry too much about this. Almost all parents do accept that they are responsible for bringing their children up adequately, but

the interpretation of adequately is infinitely variable. But how easy it is for a young unmarried doctor to criticize the way in which a young unmarried mother is raising her family!

A mistaken diagnosis of child abuse will inevitably cause much distress but the possibility often arises since the diagnosis is almost always based on probability rather than on proof (see Addy, D. P. (1985). Talking points in child abuse. *British Medical Journal*, **290**, 259–60). We must try to avoid the situation in which parents fail to avail themselves of the casualty services for the quite innocent minor injuries that children suffer (Anonymous (1981). Child abuse: the swing of the pendulum. *British Medical Journal*, **283**, 170).

Use your discretion; seek senior advice; play safe!

■ Children

About one-third of all patients seen in A & E departments are children: more children are seen there than in paediatric clinics. Dealing with injured and acutely ill children is part of the art of medicine. Experience and example can refine your basic attitudes but there is one small point of technique which is worth recording: when you first see such a child, pay no attention to his injury or illness but only to him as a person, starting with the customary greeting and moving gently on via discussion of matters of interest (clothes, toys, siblings, birthdays, etc.) to the purpose of his visit. I often find that asking a young child if he/she is married or courting or drinks beer provokes a little laughter and relieves the initial tension. But do not 'talk down' to children; talk to them, as well as to their parents.

Severe pain, of course, needs immediate relief before such courtesies begin.

A special children's waiting area should be provided and children should be dealt with as soon as reasonably possible: if an adult patient objects to this, announcing that he arrived first, I inform him of the location of other casualty departments and suggest that he takes his

ailments elsewhere. Children's cubicles should be decorated appropriately with pleasant (washable) wallpaper and mobiles and the young patients should be sheltered from the unpleasant sights and sounds as far as possible. 'Certificates of Bravery' can be awarded to deserving children. Close liaison with the paediatric department is of the greatest benefit to all concerned.

The good management of ill and injured children is, to my mind, the most rewarding aspect of Accident and Emergency work: it is not an easy skill to acquire but one well worth cultivating. Special aspects of the care of such children are admirably dealt with in Cynthia Illingworth's book: see **Bibliography**.

■ Clinical trials

The benefits to an accident unit of regularly conducting limited prospective clinical trials are immense. The patients benefit from the instant rise in interest that is generated and the staff proportionately. The practical benefits that arise are not inconsiderable either, in an area where there are wide and fundamental disparities in everyday practice. Provided that the trial is limited in its scope, and carefully designed to test the minimum of variables (two only if possible), clear and statistically significant results can be obtained which allow objective improvements in the rational care of injured patients. The accident field offers endless scope for this elementary and satisfying activity, which should be encouraged in every way possible provided that patients are helped by it without being put to unjustifiable inconvenience, and adequate supervision and control of the design and management of the trial is available.

Longer term research projects in Accident and Emergency units are of even greater value in maintaining the intellectual and scientific acumen and enthusiasm of senior staff, as well as making a potential contribution to more effective patient care. Computerization of records will produce invaluable opportunities in this field.

■ Clinics

Make sure you know what clinics are available and when. There will be a notice board somewhere in your department with the necessary details. Most hospitals have specific clinics for:

Fractures
Hand injuries
Lumps and bumps
Venereal disease

There is space opposite to record times and places.

Some consultants encourage direct referrals to specialist medical, surgical, orthopaedic, dermatological, otorhinolaryngological, or whatever clinics. Some insist on referral via the patient's own GP. Find out the policy on referrals, then act accordingly.

It is important to have routine follow-up clinics run by a senior member of staff, preferably a consultant, in order to provide a supervisory function and to keep the number of return visits to a minimum.

■ Cold injury

Cold epidermolysis

See **Blisters**

Frost-bite

Peripheral gangrene usually of fingers or toes due to prolonged circulatory shut-down and interstitial ice formation with irreversible tissue damage. A surgical problem. The slowest possible re-warming is essential.

Hypothermia (q.v.)

Trench foot

Cold immersion in mud or water without freezing produces ischaemia; re-warming causes a hyperaemic, red, and painful extremity, responding to the accumulated tissue metabolites of the ischaemic phase. If this situation is recurrent or prolonged tissue death arises.

A general recommendation is to warm ischaemic tissue dry and slowly, to cool painful hyperaemic tissue, preferably with a fan, and to avoid scrupulously any trauma to tissue-damaged areas by pressure or friction.

After the primary treatment (which is largely aimed at preventing further damage) general surgical principles prevail.

■ Collapse and coma

Collapse is an overworked label which includes all sorts of emotional upsets from terror to tantrums. Coma is a more definite condition of inaccessible loss of consciousness, but the two overlap and are more easily dealt with together.

1 Take a history from the patient and/or relatives and/or witnesses and/or ambulancemen.

2 Examine the patient fully, beginning with such fundamentals as the pulse, blood pressure, temperature, respiratory rate, pupil size and reaction, and conscious level.

3 Useful baseline investigations include the following: venous blood for full blood count including platelets, urea and electrolytes, glucose, amylase, paracetamol and salicylate levels, group and save serum; arterial blood for gases; ECG; chest X-ray and skull X-ray.

Primary care for every variety of collapse or coma consists in establishment of an airway and its maintenance; the supply of oxygen; supportive treatment, e.g. intravenous infusion and the maintenance of the heart's action. Gradually the underlying condition may become manifest as more clinical and circumstantial evidence is

accumulated (e.g. from the patient's property or previous hospital or GP notes), but generally more specific treatment is the responsibility of the receiving physician.

When trying to make a diagnosis, remember that common conditions (e.g. hypoglycaemia, hyperglycaemia, cerebrovascular accident, head injury, myocardial infarction, drunkenness, epilepsy, overdose) are more likely to occur than rarities: ruptured splenic artery aneurysm is unlikely to present more than twice each day!

Physical causes of collapse and coma include the following. Details of their treatments are given elsewhere in this book or in standard texts: see **Bibliography**. In a world of rapid travel and disturbed politics exotic diseases can turn up anywhere and every casualty officer needs to have them in his mind. For your own interest, make a list opposite of the number of causes you meet during your time in A & E.

Hypovolaemic shock due to internal or external haemorrhage

- Bleeding from the gastrointestinal tract, e.g. oesophageal varices, Mallory–Weiss syndrome, peptic ulceration, neoplasm
- Obstetrical or gynaecological causes, e.g. ruptured ectopic pregnancy, spontaneous abortion, antepartum or post-partum haemorrhage
- Traumatic haemorrhage
- Ruptured aortic aneurysm
- Blood abnormalities or dyscrasias
- Spontaneous rupture of a varicose vein: a ruptured varicose vein only needs elevation of the limb to staunch the bleeding and make surgical closure simpler
- Epistaxis

Blood volume replacement urgently with Haemaccel and then with cross-matched blood meets the emergency.

Hypovolaemic shock due to loss of fluid

- Vomiting
- Diarrhoea
- Diuresis

Hypovolaemic shock due to loss of plasma

- Burns

Cardiogenic shock

- Myocardial infarction
- Cardiac arrest
- Left ventricular failure, especially with aortic stenosis
- Dysrhythmia, especially heart block leading to Stokes–Adams attacks, but also ventricular arrhythmia and acute atrial fibrillation
- Paroxysmal tachycardia
- Cardiac tamponade
- Pulmonary embolus
- Atrial myxoma acting as intermittent ball-valve

Respiratory crises

- 'Café coronary': bolus impaction in the laryngeal introitus; treated by a series of brisk 'bear-hugs' in the epigastrium, standing behind the patient (Heimlich's manoeuvre): the foreign body is hopefully 'blown out'; infants can be held upside-down and patted on the back; in an adult, a back blow causes a foreign body in the throat to be propelled downward and backward, either impacting in the glottis or passing into the lung, Cf. **Foreign bodies.**
- Pneumothorax, spontaneous or traumatic
- Tension pneumothorax
- Subacute pneumonia in the aged
- Breath-holding attacks in infants

- Hyperventilation is often associated with syncope (vaso-vagal attacks), hysteria, and carpo-pedal spasm; treat by rebreathing the air in a paper bag or give O_2/CO_2 mixture by mask; common in unstable teenagers
- Acute bronchiolitis in small children
- Acute laryngo-tracheo-bronchitis

Neurological crises

- Cerebrovascular accident
- Subarachnoid haemorrhage
- CNS infection
- Transient ischaemic attack
- Subdural/extradural haematoma
- Cerebral neoplasm
- Vertebro-basilar insufficiency (pulpit watcher's syndrome): posture-associated syncopal attacks due to a combination of atherosclerosis and cervical spondylosis
- Epilepsy, with its puzzling post-ictal confusion

Poisoning

- Self-poisoning (including alcohol): narcotic drugs are reversed by naloxone (0.8 mg intravenously, repeated every 2 minutes as required)
- Accidental poisoning
- Carbon monoxide poisoning is now mostly found in closed garages, cars stuck in snow-drifts with their engines running to keep their occupants warm, and closed rooms with leaky stove-pipes; town gas supplies in Great Britain are now only harmful in so far as they can displace the oxygen content of a closed room and so produce asphyxia; in some other countries coal is still coked to produce carbon monoxide

Endocrine disorders

- Diabetes: hypoglycaemic coma or keto-acidosis; lactic acidosis
- Myxoedema coma
- Acute thyrotoxic crisis
- Acute hypopituitarism, e.g pituitary thrombosis following post-partum haemorrhage (pituitary apoplexy)
- Acute adrenocortical insufficiency can be due to incautious corticosteroid withdrawal or acute stress (e.g. road traffic accident) in a patient with undiagnosed adrenocortical insufficiency (borderline Addison's disease)
- Waterhouse–Friderichsen syndrome (see below)

Miscellaneous

- Trauma, especially head injury
- Uraemia: may be precipitated by infection, dehydration, or drugs in borderline renal failure
- Hepatic coma
- Hypothermia
- Hyperpyrexia: can develop in children rapidly in hot weather, especially in victims of cystic fibrosis
- Sickle cell crisis
- Hypertensive encephalopathy
- Wernicke's encephalopathy (vitamin B_1 deficiency) in alcoholics and the chronically starved
- Inanition/dehydration syndromes in the poor and neglected
- Anaphylactic shock: wasp and bee stings can produce rapidly fatal anaphylactic reactions in hypersensitive people

- Toxic shock: toxaemia from sepsis, local or general, is a first consideration especially in diabetics or people debilitated by disease or malnutrition; treatment is with an energetic combination of intravenous antibiotics and intravenous plasma substitute; the possibility of using a vasopressor drug such as dopamine should not be ruled out when collapse is life-threatening
- Acute septicaemic conditions: influenzal cardio-myopathy; meningococcal septicaemia leading to acute adrenal bleeding (Waterhouse–Friderichsen syndrome), which can also happen with other bacterial septicaemias
- Infections, including malaria, typhoid, and rabies
- Food poisoning, especially when accompanied by severe vomiting and purging; botulism is the most severe of this type and can be rapidly fatal
- Poisonous bites, scorpion and centipede stings, and jellyfish poisoning

■ Complaints

These are divisible into three types:

1 **The genuine** A mistake has occurred (e.g. a fractured scaphoid has been missed) or a member of staff has behaved unprofessionally (e.g. criticized one patient in front of another).

2 **The understandable** The patient is unhappy regarding his treatment (e.g. not being given local anaesthesia for a single suture) or its result (e.g. the residual scar after a severe laceration) or some other aspect of his visit (e.g. the time he had to wait); in fact, though, nothing has gone wrong. Sympathetic explanation almost always defuses the situation and re-establishes the favourable reputation of the department in the district; if it does not, type 2 becomes type 3.

3 **The absurd** The patient is invariably either a fool (e.g. he believes nurses should never eat or drink coffee or even laugh) or totally self-centred (e.g. he genuinely considers that he should be dealt with immediately, regardless of the fact that other patients are obviously more seriously ill or injured). It took me many years to realize the fact that many people do not worry one jot about the misfortunes of others. Never apologize to these people. Treat them correctly and as politely as you can manage and get rid of them as soon as possible. Don't let them upset you: they're just not worth it.

A few pieces of advice:

- Consult your consultant and your defence union as soon as a potentially serious situation seems possible.
- Always make good notes.
- Never criticize a colleague (medical or otherwise); criticism with the retrospectoscope but without the full facts is easy and tempting.
- When something has gone wrong, explain the facts to the patient and strive to rectify the situation sympathetically.
- Remember that everyone makes mistakes, certainly every practising doctor. Consultants know this, so do protection societies, so do your peers, and judges and coroners; even some patients accept the fact. You will make them too: recognize them when you do, and learn from them.

Cf. **Mistakes, some common**

■ Computerization of A & E records

This offers great hopes of advances in managing the vast and variable work-load of the accident and emergency services. If intelligently designed and applied with due sense of priorities it can provide an invaluable data base for clinical and epidemiological research.

■ Confusion, acute

Hypoglycaemia (q.v.) Give intravenous glucose 25–50 g; see **Diabetic emergencies**.

Epilepsy Give intravenous diazepam (Diazemuls) 5–10 mg.

Toxaemia Diagnosis and general supportive treatment are needed, especially restoration of circulating blood volume and blood pressure.

Senile degeneration Mild sedation is required and admission if necessary.

Emotional stress Elucidation is best done before sedation if possible.

Major psychiatric illness Specialist admission may be required under the relevant section of the Mental Health Act (see **Psychiatric emergencies**).

Hypoxia Especially occurs in head injuries (q.v.).

■ Convulsions, febrile

By definition, simple febrile convulsions occur in children aged between 6 months and 5 years, last less than 15 minutes, have no focal features, and leave no permanent CNS signs. Remove the child's clothes, fan him, and sponge him with cool water. Lie him semi-prone to avoid aspiration. A child who has had a prolonged convulsion may be unrousable but most can be roused.

The fits can be controlled with intravenous diazepam (Diazemuls, 0.15–0.25 mg/kg given very slowly) or rectal diazepam (Stesolid rectal tubes, one 5 mg tube below the age of 3 years, one 10 mg tube over the age of 3 years). Paraldehyde is a safe alternative; give 0.2 ml/kg by deep intramuscular injection: not more than 2 ml should be given at any one site and it should not be in a plastic syringe for longer than 2 minutes. Paraldehyde can also be given rectally: 1 ml per year of life + 1 ml, e.g. 3 ml for a 2-year-old child.

The source of the pyrexia should be sought: consider especially the meninges, chest, ears, throat, and urine. Take blood samples for culture and glucose levels. Most of these children have a generalized viral infection. Most do not need an antibiotic. Paracetamol (120–250 mg 4-hourly as needed) will lower the temperature.

A first febrile convulsion should usually be admitted; others should be discussed with a paediatrician before being allowed home.

■ Cot death

Cot death (Sudden Infant Death Syndrome) is the commonest cause of death in infants aged between 4 weeks and 1 year. One baby in every 500 live births dies suddenly, silently and unexpectedly, for no obvious reason. The tragedy is world-wide. Parental shock and bewilderment are devastating and long-lasting; they frequently experience feelings of guilt, quite unfounded. The peak incidence is at 2–5 months of age but infants up to 2 years old can be affected.

In the Accident and Emergency department, death is confirmed and any obvious cause (e.g. trauma) is eliminated by external examination. Breaking the dreadful news to the parents is overwhelmingly difficult; explain that the death appears to be a cot death but that baby has not suffered at all. After a little while, the parents must be allowed to see and cuddle their baby (clothed) and say good-bye before baby is taken to the mortuary; they will require privacy for this, though they may welcome the company of a sympathetic nurse.

Explain that the coroner will need to be informed and that a post-mortem examination will be required.

Inform, as soon as possible, the paediatric team, the General Practitioner and the coroner's officer. A hospital chaplain often brings comfort and support; the parents may wish the child to be baptized. Others who may need to be informed include the health visitor and the social worker.

Ensure that continued support is arranged for the parents. The mother, if breast-feeding, will need immediate advice on the suppression of lactation. It may be necessary to make arrangements for the care of siblings.

The bereaved parents should be given a copy of the very helpful leaflet *Information for parents following the sudden and unexpected death of their baby.* This is published by The Foundation for the Study of Infant Deaths, 5th Floor, 4 Grosvenor Place, London SW1X 7HD (01-235-1721 or 01-245-9421). Copies should be kept in the department and you should read it yourself. The Foundation also publishes *Guidelines for accident and emergency departments.*

Staff training is helpful in learning to manage this catastrophe. A senior doctor should always be involved from the outset.

■ Croup

See **Stridor, acute**

■ Dental, miscellaneous

Bleeding extraction site

1 Tell the patient to bite on a dental roll for at least 45 minutes.
2 Give intravenous tranexamic acid (Cyklokapron) 0.5–1 g slowly, followed by oral tranexamic acid 1 g three times a day for 48 hours.
3 Pack with absorbable haemostatic gauze (Surgicel) or an adrenaline pack.
4 If no good, oversew the socket with 3/0 Dexon.
5 Prescribe broad-spectrum antibiotics.
6 Remember the possibility of blood dyscrasia or anticoagulant therapy.

Toothache

Patients should be referred to a dentist at the earliest convenient opportunity. Prescribe analgesia as required, and broad-spectrum antibiotics if there is an abscess (detected by swelling and tenderness on tapping the tooth). Refer immediately if the abscess is pointing extra-orally.

Dental injury

Patients with chipped teeth should be referred to a dentist: immediately if the pulp is exposed. Patients with displaced teeth should be referred immediately. Avulsed teeth should be placed in normal saline: they can be successfully re-implanted by a dentist if this is done within a few hours.

Cf. **Fractures, maxillo-facial injuries**

■ Diabetic emergencies

Hypoglycaemia is common and urgent. The patient is often restless, aggressive and pale. Deterioration is rapid and leads to coma. There is tachycardia and sweating and fits may develop.

- Take blood for glucose level
- Give 50–100 ml of 50% dextrose intravenously (proportionately less for children) and observe for at least 2 hours after consciousness is regained
- Give further carbohydrate as circumstances suggest
- Admit children and any patients likely to require stabilization

Hyperglycaemic ketoacidosis develops more gradually (over a few days); the patient becomes dehydrated, acidotic, and comatose; he hyperventilates and his breath smells ketotic.

- Take blood for glucose, urea and electrolytes, and full blood count
- Take arterial blood for gases
- Set up an intravenous infusion of 0.9% saline: 1.5 l/h initially for adults, proportionately less for children
- Admit the patient urgently under the care of the physicians or paediatricians, who will give insulin by infusion or intramuscularly, and will monitor the patient carefully, both clinically and biochemically.

■ Dislocations

Whereas fractures can usually be reduced at the earliest convenient opportunity (assuming there is no arterial obstruction or other urgent problem), dislocations are best reduced as soon as possible: the longer they are left, the more difficult they are to reduce.

The key to successful reduction is good muscle relaxation. Midazolam (Hypnovel) is excellent; the usual dose is 70 μg/kg by slow intravenous injection, until the patient becomes drowsy. Draw up 10 mg and inject very slowly, keeping the patient talking as you press the plunger; as soon as conversation begins to die away, stop injecting: the usual dose range is 2.5–7.5 mg (2.5 mg may be sufficient in elderly patients). It is a good muscle-relaxant and has a shorter half-life than diazepam, and consequently a shorter recovery period. Post-operative amnesia is excellent. There have been reports of respiratory depression (sometimes associated with hypotension), so oxygen and equipment for intubation and resuscitation must be readily available. Patients should be accompanied home by a responsible adult and should not drive or operate machinery for 8 hours.

General anaesthesia may be needed, especially if large joints (e.g. hip or shoulder) are dislocated in muscular young patients.

Always X-ray the joint after reduction, even if only for medico-legal reasons. Refer to fracture clinic for follow-up after reduction.

Notable dislocations include the following.

Ankle and foot

Usually in association with fractures, but simple dislocations can occur.

Knee

May be anterior or posterior; both can occlude the popliteal artery and both need urgent reduction.

Patella

Easy to reduce with firm pressure on its lateral aspect. The easier the reduction, the more likely is recurrence of the dislocation: surgery is sometimes required for recurrent dislocation. A plaster of Paris cylinder is advisable for six weeks after a first dislocation; if there have been previous episodes, apply a pressure bandage for 1 or 2 weeks. Build up the quads.

Hip

Usually posterior, with its characteristic deformity of adduction, internal rotation, slight flexion, and extreme pain. Test for sciatic nerve involvement. A concurrent fracture of the acetabular margin may produce instability of the reduction. Reduction is best achieved with general anaesthesia, the patient lying on the floor. The surgeon stands over him holding the leg with 90° hip and knee flexion. An assistant steadies the pelvis. Upwards traction achieves reduction with a 'clunk'. Open reduction is sometimes needed, but can generally be avoided if a muscle relaxant is given by the anaesthetist.

Anterior dislocations and central fracture-dislocations also occur.

Pelvis

Major pelvic dislocation at symphysis or sacro-iliac joint is generally part of a severe or multiple pelvic injury. Urinary complications must be considered. Major blood loss accompanies this injury.

Phalanges or digits

One sharp longitudinal tweak; no anaesthetic, or a digital nerve block. Sometimes reduction is impossible, suggesting that the head of the proximal bone has 'button-holed' through the capsule of the joint: open reduction may be necessary. Metacarpophalangeal dislocation of the thumb may need open reduction with division of the collateral ligament(s); these then need repair.

Dislocated lunate

This is easily overlooked, so always specifically examine the lunate when studying an X-ray of the wrist: the lateral view shows the cup of the lunate (normally filled with the capitate) to be empty and facing anteriorly; the antero-posterior view shows the lunate as triangular, rather than its normal quadrilateral shape. Examine for signs of median nerve involvement. Missing the diagnosis can have very serious consequences (e.g. difficulty in reduction; avascular necrosis). Reduce by extension and traction, followed by pressure on the lunate and flexion. Apply plaster of Paris in flexion.

Elbow

Look for damage to the artery or nerves. A helper applies traction at the wrist (elbow at 90°); the surgeon applies firm pressure over the olecranon with two thumbs. Avoid passive movement in the weeks after injury, to reduce the chances of myositis ossificans.

Pulled elbow

A commonly encountered problem is for an infant or child, less than 5 years old, to be brought 'not using his arm'. Classically the history is of a traction injury (e.g. being swung by his parents while walking) but this is far from invariable; frequently the only obtainable story is that the child has fallen. Presumably the pathology is a distal subluxation of the radial head in the annular ligament.

The child is miserable and the arm is held limply and unused, because pronation/supination cause pain. Begin by examining the clavicle and shoulder area: fractures of the clavicle or proximal humerus are common. Next examine the forearm, wrist and hand: greenstick fractures of the distal radius are again frequent. Having excluded these, examine the shaft and distal humerus and gently flex and extend the elbow, eliminating supracondylar injuries.

Thus far, the child has whimpered. Now hold the child's hand (with your left hand if his left arm is injured and right for right) and his elbow with your other hand and, with the elbow at right angles, push the hand proximally, simultaneously pronating and supinating the forearm. A distinct click is felt at the elbow, the child shrieks but, usually within 5 minutes, he is using the arm normally again. I allow him home once he can put both hands on his head or pick up a sweet with the injured arm. If this is a recurrent episode, give him an 'inescapable' collar-and-cuff for a few days.

X-rays are of no value, unless this manoeuvre fails to provide relief.

Shoulder

An anterior dislocation is much the commonest: reduce by Kocher's method, but test sensation to pin-prick in the axillary nerve area first. Kocher's method of reduction consists of 4 consecutive manoeuvres:

1   traction on the flexed elbow for 3 or 4 minutes;
2   external rotation of the arm;
3   adduction of the arm;
4   internal rotation of the arm.

If reduction is unsuccessful using midazolam, try again under general anaesthesia. After reduction, a patient with a first or second dislocation should wear a broad arm sling under the clothes for four weeks, to reduce the risk of recurrent dislocation; if the shoulder has been dislocated a few times before, simply rest the arm for a few days and consider reconstructive surgery. Mobilize elderly patients early to avoid stiffness.

An associated fracture of the greater tuberosity usually reduces well with the dislocation but may need open reduction. Dislocation of the shoulder with a fracture of the surgical neck of the humerus usually needs operative reduction.

Posterior dislocation of the shoulder is unusual and easily missed, because the anteroposterior X-ray often appears to be normal: but check whether the surfaces of the humeral head and the glenoid are congruent. If the shoulder is painful, tender, and deformed, obtain a lateral X-ray and study it very carefully.

Acromioclavicular joint

Dislocation of the acromioclavicular joint can be treated with a sling, worn until the pain subsides (Anonymous (1986). Acromioclavicular dislocations: conservative treatment vindicated. *Lancet*, **ii**, 1079).

Jaw

Dislocation is always anterior when spontaneous (due to yawning, laughing, etc.). To replace, give intravenous midazolam—sufficient to produce calm and relaxation—then stand facing the seated patient; apply your thumbs to his mandible each side behind the last molar; press downwards, while lifting the angle of the jaw forwards and upwards with your fingers. Your reduction will be successful. Apply the standard first-aid bandage to prevent redislocation.

■ Drowning

In hospital, treat as you would asphyxia of any other kind:

- Airway
- Intubation if necessary
- Tracheal suction
- Cardiac resuscitation
- Serum electrolytes measurement
- Admission

Patients, especially children, can survive after prolonged periods of submersion in water.

Aspiration of water into the lungs may result in the adult respiratory distress syndrome (acute pulmonary oedema with normal left atrial pressure) within 24 hours: 'secondary drowning'.

Positive end expiratory pressure (PEEP) respiration may be required if pulmonary (and cerebral) oedema develop as late complications of near-drowning. Cerebral oedema can be reduced by slow rewarming and mechanical hyperventilation.

Cf. **Hypothermia**

■ Drug addiction

A familiar problem in urban A & E units. The primary condition is not our responsibility but secondary effects may be, e.g. infection, acute psychiatric disorder, withdrawal syndromes, self-injury, and numerous associated psychopathic manifestations of manipulative kinds aimed at securing drug supplies. Encephalopathies occur in glue-sniffers as well as alcoholics. Disposal is a major problem.

Cf. **Psychiatric emergencies**

■ Drunkenness

The acutely drunk who are injured (and too often injure others) offer special problems: the diagnosis of their injuries is clouded by their drunkenness at every turn; they are difficult to handle and may assault staff, especially if they sense that staff are unsure of themselves; they are difficult to treat because they are irrational, unco-operative, and sometimes vomiting. The largest problem is to make sure whether they are just drunk, or drunk and ill, or drunk and injured. If you are in doubt, keep them under observation, preferably on the floor where they cannot fall any further. Protect the airway: try to keep them in the coma position. If you have no doubt that they are merely drunk, ask the police to cope. In the increasingly awkward medico-legal climate in Western countries routine blood alcohol estimations (strictly confidential) give some protection to the casualty officer accused of negligence. They are also of value clinically in assessing the severity of concomitant head injury. Measure the blood sugar if the patient is unresponsive, to detect hypoglycaemia. To avoid Korsakov's psychosis, intravenous Parentrovite should be given before intravenous dextrose (50 ml of 50%) if the patient is thought to be a chronic alcoholic.

Delirium tremens is a psychiatric emergency and to be treated as such, i.e. by certification, without sedation if possible. It is an acute withdrawal mania.

Cf. **Psychiatric emergencies**

Dysphagia

A term used properly to describe difficult swallowing and improperly (but with equal frequency) to describe inability to swallow, or oesophageal occlusion (q.v.). True dysphagia is not really an A & E problem.

Ear, nose, and throat emergencies

It has been said that there is only one ENT emergency, namely sudden perceptive deafness due to viral acoustic neuropathy, which requires urgent treatment with steroids, but some of the laryngeal crises and upper oesophageal calamities qualify as well.

Cf. **Epistaxis; Asphyxia; Oesophageal occlusion; Fractures, maxillo-facial injuries**

Ears

Foreign bodies

Remove under direct vision if possible; general anaesthetic may be required. Avoid trauma; avoid pushing further into the ear; use oil; give antibiotics. Syringing in the presence of trauma or occlusion often does more harm than good. Use a loop or blunt hook, skill, and experience. Suction may be helpful.

Insects

Drown with warm olive oil or liquid paraffin before removal by forceps or syringe.

Otitis externa

Use gentle toilet and antibiotic eardrops (e.g. Otosporin). If very painful and swollen, glycerine and ichthammol help a lot, applied by a very gentle insertion of well-soaked gauze 1 cm wide.

Otitis media

This is a common cause of disability in young children. If severe and painful, and if there is a bulging eardrum, the need of myringotomy should be borne in mind. Antibiotics should be given in any case: amoxycillin or cephradine are suitable.

Pinna

Lacerations Careful approximation of skin edges is important, using fine (5/0 or 6/0) sutures. It is important not to stitch through the cartilage as a cauliflower ear may ensue if you do.

Haematoma Aspirate completely and apply a pressure bandage to avoid cauliflower ear. The bandage (crêpe or Tubigrip) goes over a thick (2.5 cm), soft, sterile foam pad. Aspiration may have to be repeated several times, and a small instillation of methylprednisolone (Depo-Medrone, 0.5 ml) may reduce the ultimate scarring. This is a difficult and time-consuming procedure, but untreated haematoma gives a horrible deformity. If haematoma involves the cartilage of the pinna itself it may need incision and drainage (fenestration) through the posterior surface. Antibiotic cover is required. When in doubt seek help from a plastic surgeon. A complicating seroma needs referral.

Haematotympanum Traumatic; usually associated with fracture of the floor of the tympanic cavity or of the petrous temporal bone itself. First aid: intramuscular antibiotics and analgesia. Specialist referral is advised.

■ Elbow

Acute tennis elbow

Frequently presents as an injury because of its acutely painful response to minor trauma. It is sometimes called non-traumatic lateral epicondylitis of the elbow. Primary treatment with rest in a sling for 10 days with a non-steroidal anti-inflammatory drug by mouth is often effective. If not, local injection of 1% lignocaine and 0.5 ml of methylprednisolone (Depo-Medrone) is usually helpful.

Cf. **Tenosynovitis**

A similar condition occurring medially is sometimes met and is called **golfer's elbow**.

Traumatic synovitis of the elbow

Commonly ensues after falls on the outstretched hand or directly on the elbow without X-ray evidence of injury to bone. It should always be treated by rest in a sling and patience. It may recover very slowly (10 days to 4 weeks) and should never be hurried. Hand and shoulder movements *must* be maintained throughout this tiresome period of recovery.

See also **Dislocations** and **Fractures, upper limb**

■ Emergencies, miscellaneous

Non-cardiac chest pain

This condition may present with much anxiety. *Pectoral myalgia* (with superficial tenderness) is common; *Tietze's disease* (osteochondritis of one or more costochondral junctions) responds to local infiltration with bupivacaine and methylprednisolone acetate (Depo-Medrone) 40 mg.

Cf. **Myocardial infarction**, *pseudo-coronary*

Perianal haematoma (thrombotic external pile)

Simple incision under local anaesthesia and evacuation of the clot gives relief.

See also **Injuries, minor**

■ Endocrine emergencies

These do not commonly present in A & E units but have to be borne in mind in the differential diagnosis of **Collapse and coma** (q.v.). They include:

- Thyrotoxic crisis
- Hyperthyroid cardiac failure
- Myxoedema coma (elderly patients) especially in cold weather
- Waterhouse–Friderichsen syndrome (adrenal haemorrhage)
- Phaeochromocytoma with paroxysmal hypertension
- Pituitary coma
- Pituitary apoplexy
- Addison's disease

Thyrotoxic crisis

This can present with a variety of symptoms, including irritability, confusion, delirium, hyperpyrexia, tachycardia, diarrhoea, and eye-rolling. Propranolol 5–10 mg intravenously controls flutter; acute fibrillation requires digitalization. Give hydrocortisone 100 mg intravenously and treat other symptoms as necessary — e.g. cooling with fans and damp sheets for hyperpyrexia; intravenous diazepam provides sedation. Refer to the physicians.

Myxoedema coma

This occurs in hypothyroid people particularly in cold weather. They need tri-iodothyronine 10 μg intravenously, hydrocortisone, and standard treatment for **Hypothermia** (q.v.), and should be admitted to the intensive therapy unit.

Addisonian crisis

This is characterized by shock, hypotension, hypoglycaemia, stupor, and terminal coma. It is usually seen in known cases of Addison's disease and meningococcal septicaemia (cf. **Collapse and coma**). Treatment is intravenous dextrose-saline and hydrocortisone 100 mg. Transfer to the intensive therapy unit after taking blood for baseline electrolyte measurements.

■ Endotracheal intubation

This procedure takes practice (Scott, D. B. (1986). Endotracheal intubation: friend or foe. *British Medical Journal*, **292**, 157–8). You need to be able to do it instantly in every case in whom it is needed. An anaesthetist is the best teacher, but an intubation model is a good second best.

Prolonged intubation needs a clear plastic tube with the balloon moderately inflated. Measure the distance from the incisors to the cricoid and trim the tube so that it will lie comfortably with the connector at the lips and the balloon 2–3 cm below the vocal cords. If the tube is too long you may occlude the left main bronchus with consequent collapse of the lung.

Intubation is the paramount life-saving technique of the casualty officer. Positive pressure ventilation can be maintained indefinitely using an ordinary anaesthetic apparatus or an Ambu bag with an appropriate connector.

Epiglottitis

See **Stridor, acute**

Epistaxis

Treat by:
1 Digital compression, for 10 minutes.
2 Sedation and rest for the agitated, in a position of comfort and drainage.
3 If these simple remedies are ineffective give intravenous tranexamic acid (Cyklokapron) 0.5–1 g slowly, followed by oral tranexamic acid 1 g three times a day for 48 hours.
4 This remedy has a high success rate, but occasionally the elderly arteriosclerotic or hypertensive patient needs nasal packing. Use either bismuth oxide paste ribbon-gauze or ribbon-gauze soaked in liquid paraffin. Nasal packing *must* be done properly. If you do not know how, ask someone who does to show you. It is built up, fold upon fold, with 2.5 cm ribbon-gauze until the cavity is *lightly* filled.
5 Very rarely an acute necrotizing rhinitis can bring about an epistaxis which proves fatal if untreated. This may well require ligation of both maxillary and both anterior ethmoidal arteries. I hope you never meet one.

Epistaxis is occasionally the presenting symptom of:

- Leukaemia
- Mononucleosis
- Thrombocytopenia
- Clotting and bleeding diseases (see **Haematological emergencies**)

■ Extramural agencies

Community nurses

Available for dressings at home when distance or disability make hospital attendance difficult. Community nurses have a high standard of practice, but are pretty thin on the ground.

Social workers

Often difficult to get hold of but in theory always available somewhere to deal with problems such as accommodation, financial aid, certification of the insane, child abuse, and family difficulties. They tend to get blamed for not producing the answers for the mass of psychopaths and sociopaths that are handed on to them.

They are human and have an uncertain role in society, being in some doubt whether their obligation is primarily to their 'clients', or to the social organization as a whole.

Ambulance staff

Ambulance staff give a high standard of first aid *en route* and are good assessors, usually, of the seriousness of injuries. Patients with major or multiple injuries often need many hands for lifting, undressing, and splinting; ambulance crews are experienced and willing helpers on arrival. Accident departments have an obligation to maintain the interest and standards of training of ambulance staff, who respond enthusiastically to discussion, being asked for evidence, instruction, and general inclusion in the accident 'family'.

Police

Uniformly helpful but limited by legal considerations. Violent, disturbed, or inebriated characters who show signs of physical aggression and do not yield to the blandishments of charming nursing staff are often calmed by a police presence. Police and accident staff meet very often and have much to give each other. You need to help them if you want them to help you. The police share with A & E staff the dubious distinction of becoming involved when an individual is suddenly in difficulties and therefore feels threatened; consequently we both tend to endure much unnecessary abuse, and to appreciate each other's difficulties. Problems of confidentiality of information about patients sometimes cause misunderstanding: frank and honest discussion generally resolves them, as police are just as anxious as the rest of us to keep doctor/patient communications confidential.

■ Eyes

Chemosis, acute

See **Hay fever**

Corneal abrasions

Common in windy weather, gardeners, and people who put their heads out of carriage windows. If blepharospasm is so severe as to prevent examination, instil two drops of amethocaine 1% into the conjunctival sac and then examine with a good light before and after instilling fluorescein drops: an abrasion shows a fixed green fluorescence. If there is any corneal damage it should be treated with chloramphenicol 1% ointment, and a pad and bandage, and referred to an ophthalmologist if not healed within 2 or 3 days. If amethocaine has been used, the patient must wear an eye pad for 6 hours, as the normal corneal reflex is temporarily lost.

Corneal foreign bodies

If superficial, these can be easily removed with the side of a 23 G needle after local anaesthesia with two drops of 1% amethocaine. The corneal integrity should be tested with fluorescein afterwards, and treated as above if not intact. Chemicals in the eye need copious irrigation. Again, an eye pad is required for 6 hours if amethocaine has been used.

Eye injuries

All injuries to the lacrimal apparatus, tarsal plates, and full thickness injuries of the lids need the urgent opinion of an ophthalmologist. Major injuries to the globe of the eye need early assessment and treatment, often at the same time as associated multiple injuries. Send every hyphaema to the specialist. Send urgently for expert ophthalmic advice in cases of lacerations of the cornea or sclera, ocular concussion, or any other eye injury involving internal bleeding or external vitreous leakage.

Swollen, contused eyes and ordinary oedematous black eyes need antibiotic eye ointment until normal drainage is re-established.

X-ray the orbit for foreign bodies if there is any risk of these, particularly if the injury occurred when hammering.

Orbital 'blow-out' injury

In association with maxillary fracture involving the floor of the orbit this can lead to entrapment of the inferior rectus muscle. Warning signs are painful limitation of eye elevation and infraorbital sensory loss. This is an ophthalmic emergency requiring operative release of the entrapped muscle if permanent ophthalmoplegia is to be avoided. Tomography of the orbit is useful for diagnosis.

Orbital emphysema/pneumatocoele

See **Fractures, maxillo-facial injuries**

■ Facial lacerations

Primary suture by experienced and painstaking accident staff has much to offer. Plastic surgeons can offer little in addition unless the lacerations are associated with structural damage (see **Fractures, maxillo-facial injuries**), or with skin loss needing emergency grafting operations.

The tiny, raised, often semi-lunar lacerations made by glass spicules should be excised and sutured with the finest non-absorbable sutures if the patient's condition warrants it. If not stitched they cause disfigurement.

Look for damage to facial nerves, nasolacrimal, and parotid ducts.

Gravel rash of the face needs 10 minutes scrubbing under general anaesthesia.

■ Fish bones

In the pharynx or oesophagus. The following pointers are useful in deciding if there really is a significant bone present:

● What kind of fish? For example, cod bones are dangerous, kipper bones are not.
● Was the meal finished?
● Is the pain localized?
● Can the patient swallow, without grimacing, (a) water, (b) dry bread?

Do a careful inspection of the tonsils and pharynx, and an indirect pharyngoscopy and laryngoscopy; fine bones often stick into the pharyngeal or lingual tonsil. Give a large dose of intramuscular ampicillin and review in the morning. If there is severe pain and muscle spasm, or a positive radiograph, inform the ENT department and admit, especially so if there is pooling of saliva in the piriform fossae. Removal of non-opaque bones demonstrated by Gastrografin swallow may be required as an emergency. If you are in much doubt refer for oesophagoscopy.

The same applies, of course, to other kinds of bones as well, but these are generally radio-opaque and so easier to assess.

■ Fish hooks

These have to be removed in the direction of entry because of the barb. Inject 1 ml of lignocaine under the hook; cut the shank with wire-cutters below the eye; seize the shank with a needle-holder, push the point of the hook onwards through the skin, and remove.

An alternative method is to push the barb through the skin, cut it off, and then withdraw the hook shank first.

■ Food poisoning

Not a common A & E presentation, but the more dramatic forms may cause problems by their very unfamiliarity.

Botulism

Intoxication by *Clostridium botulinum* in tinned food, characterized by prostration and severe myasthenia after 8–24 hours of nausea and vomiting; assisted respiration may be required because of respiratory neuromuscular block; antitoxin should be given intravenously as soon as the diagnosis is made.

Salmonella food poisoning

Commonly due to *Salmonella typhimurium*, through rodent contamination of food; presents as a communal, febrile gastro-enteritis.

Staphylococcal food poisoning

Due to staphylococcal infection of food handlers: rapid onset and an afebrile course with early prostration.

Primary care of salmonella and staphylococcal food poisoning lies simply in rehydration and then supportive treatment.

Acute infective diarrhoeas

These can present as emergencies. Prolonged diarrhoea with fever, bloody stools, or toxaemic collapse demands investigation. First treatment is the same for all: intravenous rehydration. Admit. Salmonella, shigella, campylobacter, *Escherichia coli, Vibrio cholerae*, amoebiasis, and giardiasis are among the infective organisms and conditions. Physicians will sort them out.

■ Foreign bodies

Swallowed

Children will swallow anything, and what they can swallow they can almost always pass safely, regardless of shape or sharpness. There can be no justification for serial radiography to 'follow the course of a foreign object through the digestive tract'. This exposes the child to a dose of radiation which gives him or her no benefit, however much it may reassure anxious parents or cowardly doctors.

The routine is:

1 Tell the parents of the almost infinite adaptability of the infant gut.
2 Explain that radiography does not cure, or alleviate, or determine a course of action.
3 Require them to give a normal or bulky diet and to examine the stools carefully for 5 days following the ingestion, or until the object is passed: expected time of arrival is up to 5 days.
4 Abdominal pain should be reported to the GP, who must, of course, be kept in the picture.

5   If the object is not passed after five days it is justifiable to take a single straight film of the abdomen to give some idea of the progress of the journey. If the object is seen in the colon further patience is all that is needed. If it is still in the stomach, a surgical opinion should be sought.

Button batteries used in calculators, etc. may be swallowed. Usually observation is all that is required but if the battery lodges in the oesophagus, urgent intervention is necessary; a chest X-ray should be obtained, as the size of the battery is the most important factor in determining whether it will pass beyond the oesophagus; blood mercury concentrations should be measured (Kiely, B. and Gill, D. (1986). Ingestion of button batteries: hazards and management. *British Medical Journal*, **293**, 308–9).

Inhaled

These present an entirely different problem and should always be relentlessly localized and treated as a paediatric emergency *even in the absence of symptoms*. Inhalation of a foreign body is always associated with some cough or choking effect. They can cause acute respiratory distress if impacted in the larynx, and can necessitate laryngostomy. They can lodge in one of the paralaryngeal recesses and cause chronic inflammation, and eventually acute laryngeal obstruction. They can get past the larynx and cause segmental collapse of the lungs, bronchiectasis, lung abscess, and all the associated sequelae. X-ray the neck and chest and admit.

Laryngeal impaction

It is rare for this condition to be seen in an accident unit as it has generally been dealt with by an enterprising bystander or proved fatal. If it occurs in small children it is best to pick the child up by the ankles and give a smart blow between the shoulder blades. For practical reasons a different approach in large children and adults is needed. The Heimlich manoeuvre consists of delivering a sharp punch to the epigastrium in the midline so that an

explosive force is built up in the chest sufficient to clear the larynx of obstruction (Anonymous (1976). Food choking and the "Heimlich maneuver". *British Medical Journal*, **i**, 855–6).

Cf. **Collapse and coma**

Nasal

Often known or suspected by parents but may present in small children simply as unilateral, foul, nasal discharge. Removal with nasal forceps, blunt hook, or loop after adequate suction is simple under general anaesthesia; or in the conscious child if properly held by experienced nursing staff. *Rhinolith* is a rare outcome; being generally adherent it needs surgical removal.

Rectal

Almost invariably the input of sexual deviation. They need general anaesthesia and an experienced rectal surgeon as some of them do inevitable damage as they make their invariably dramatic exit.

Vaginal

Commonly a forgotten tampon, but others are sometimes inserted for sexual pleasure. Removal is usually simple. Self-abortion using a knitting needle may penetrate the posterior fornix with very serious results.

Subungual

Splinters under the nails are best removed with splinter forceps under digital nerve block; it may be necessary to remove some or all of the nail.

Foreign bodies in the soft tissues

These should be removed if they can be felt or seen. If local anaesthesia is used, infiltrate proximally, otherwise a previously palpable object may become impalpable because of the resultant swelling. A radio-opaque foreign body (metal and most glass) can be located on X-ray. If small and deep it is probably best to prescribe a course of prophylactic wide-spectrum antibiotics and leave the object in place, unless complications develop, such as infection (which makes removal easier) or tenderness. Larger and more superficial objects should generally be removed, under image-intensifier if necessary; give a course of antibiotics afterwards, if you think it advisable. Each situation should be judged on its merits but, above all, do not do further damage by cutting nerves, vessels, tendons, etc. The removal of foreign bodies from the soft tissues can be extremely difficult: you will find this out for yourself one day, if you don't believe me now.

■ Fractures, general remarks

It is clearly impossible to give a comprehensive survey of fractures and dislocations (q.v.) in a short handbook and many excellent textbooks are devoted to the subject (see **Bibliography**). However, one or two guidelines may be of service. Orthopaedic practice is subject to a large measure of personal variation, so you will need to alter these observations to suit your locality. If your department deals with several orthopaedic surgeons you will probably find that they have different requirements for the same injuries.

It is the function of the accident department to give primary treatment of adequate scope and sufficient skill to all fractures. If you are not happy about any particular case, seek the early advice of a senior clinician. It is impossible to overemphasize the importance of specialist orthopaedic care, from the beginning, for all cases of bone and joint injury. It is clearly impossible for an orthopaedic surgeon to deal personally with every such

case arriving in the accident department, but each remains primarily an orthopaedic responsibility. It is our job to treat all cases according to orthopaedic opinion and advice so that they arrive at the ward or fracture clinic appropriately sorted, supported, and comforted. Many fractures can be definitively treated at first attendance and referred to the fracture clinic for specialist supervision. A few require specialist treatment from the start. All significant fractures must be referred for specialist consideration early enough for surgical intervention if needed.

Skill in reading X-ray films is partly the fruit of experience, but still more of being careful to the point of being pernickety. If you are in doubt about a particular bone, trace the outline of each of its constituent parts with a pencil point. You won't miss many fractures. If in doubt about odd bits of bone, X-ray both sides. Ultimately clinical symptoms and signs are the determining factor, rather than radiological appearances, which are at best distorted shadows.

Children's fractures differ from those in adults in a number of respects:

- Always consider the possibility of non-accidental injury, especially in infants. Cf. **Child abuse**.
- Epiphyses can make X-ray interpretation difficult, particularly around the elbow joint: comparison views are useful; so are anatomy books.
- Greenstick fractures are easily missed on X-ray; they are usually visible on the antero-posterior view, but the lateral view shows a definite abnormal angle in the bone; as with an adult fracture, the point of tenderness is well-localized.
- The epiphysis itself can slip or fracture; subsequent growth may be arrested or uneven, with ultimate shortening or deformity.
- Healing is more rapid; in some ways this is advantageous, but there is correspondingly less time for successful intervention if required.
- Callus is particularly prominent, requiring parental reassurance.

● Remodelling can be very effective, but great expertise is needed to decide whether or not a particular angulation at a particular age is acceptable.

Pathological fractures may be secondary to malignant deposits, benign bone tumours such as chondroma, solitary cyst or fibrous dysplasia, Paget's disease in the elderly, osteogenesis imperfecta, or senile or steroidal osteoporosis. These are all common. Von Recklinghausen's disease, myeloma, haemangioma, osteoclastoma, rickets, and scurvy can also cause fractures but are rare. Primary malignant tumours rarely present as fractures.

Osteogenic sarcoma may present as a swollen and tender metaphysis; characteristic X-ray appearances identify it; in the early stages it is sometimes referred for physiotherapy, leading to tragic delay.

Fractures, maxillo-facial injuries

Ensure the airway is clear.

Mandible

Undisplaced unilateral fractures are generally untreated or given a supporting bandage. Displaced bilateral fractures need wiring. If in doubt contact the maxillo-facial surgeons. Careful X-ray studies to localize fractures in relation to dental roots are important; if you are in doubt get an orthopantomogram done.

Nasal septum

When displaced, these fractures should be referred to an ENT surgeon for assessment on about the fifth day (when the swelling has subsided). Reduction is advised for cosmetic reasons and to avoid an embarrassed airway.

Nasal bones

When fractured and much depressed require similar referral for cosmetic surgery.

Other facial bones (zygoma, maxilla, and floor of orbit)

X-rays are difficult to assess: trace the outlines of the bones and compare the two sides; inequality of radio-lucency of the two maxillary antra suggests that the denser of the two may be filled with blood, in turn suggesting a fracture of its walls. Tomography of the orbit is necessary if a 'blow-out' fracture is suspected (fracture of the floor of the orbit may lead to herniation of orbital contents with consequent ophthalmoplegia). See **Eyes**.

A depressed malar fracture is very disfiguring and needs expert handling in its reduction and maintenance. Specialist assessment should be sought in case operative reduction is required.

Extensive facial fractures (varieties of 'dish-face') need internal reduction and complicated external splintage. The Le Fort classification of maxillo-facial fractures is traditional but most facio-maxillary surgeons prefer 'upper, middle, or lower third' divisions.

Clinical signs or symptoms of facial fractures include the following:

- Palpable step (often masked by rapid swelling)
- Depression of the cheek (ditto)
- Localized tenderness
- Abnormal mobility
- Subconjunctival haemorrhage with no posterior limit
- Periorbital haematoma
- Infraorbital anaesthesia or paraesthesia
- Abnormal dental sensation
- Surgical emphysema of the orbit (orbital pneumatocoele)
- Limitation of eye movements
- Diplopia
- Blurred vision
- Enophthalmos (suggesting a 'blow-out' fracture)

- Difficulty in opening or closing the mouth
- Malocclusion
- Unilateral epistaxis

■ Fractures, neck

Fractures of the cervical spine are important and, as far as atlas and axis are concerned, can be difficult to spot. They include the majority of unstable spinal injuries. When in doubt apply a soft collar firmly and get expert advice urgently. If an unstable fracture is suspected or certain, stabilize the head with sandbags or cushions. If the radiographer can get the patient to flex the cervical spine for X-ray purposes there is not likely to be a significant fracture. Any attempt at flexion where an unstable fracture is suspected is absolutely contra-indicated. Oblique views may help to show facetal fractures or displacements.

Major neurological involvement is generally obvious. In paraplegic or tetraplegic cases, fix the head with sandbags and send for help. It is essential to look at a lateral radiograph of the neck before permitting any movement for further views. It is not rare to see tetraplegic patients after injury with no evidence of fracture on X-ray. The dynamic situation in the cervical spine is very different from the static one after the disruptive forces have ceased. Every unconscious head injury should have a 'single shot' lateral X-ray of the cervical spine before manipulation of the neck (e.g. for intubation or undressing).

Fractures, spine

Flexion injuries are common. Antero-posterior wedging is the commoner, but look for lateral wedging too. Fractures of the transverse and spinous processes are easily missed; they can be very painful but are not important in themselves, although at the upper lumbar level they may be associated with kidney damage. Unstable fractures, e.g. of the pedicles or articular processes, need handling with great respect, as described in standard texts. Careful neurological examination is essential. Uncomplicated fractures require rest until the pain subsides.

Fractures, ribs

See **Chest injuries**

Fractures, pelvis

In young people this is generally a severe injury due to major car or horse accidents. There is often visceral involvement (bladder, urethra, vagina, or rectum) and admission is required. Blood loss is often severe and replacement is usually needed. The urine must always be tested for blood and a catheter passed only on the direct instructions of the surgeon responsible. Cf. **Urogenital injuries**.

In the elderly, fracture of the pelvis is usually due to a fall and is very common. Either the ischial or pubic ramus is involved: sometimes both. Treatment consists of 10 days in bed, with leg exercises, and if the patient has good support at home admission is not required.

■ Fractures, upper limb

Clavicle

Sometimes routinely treated with a figure-of-eight bandage and broad arm sling; more usually by sling alone. Often a minor injury in children. (Obviously an occasion for a prospective clinical trial.)

Scapula

Unless so gross as to require open reduction, a broad arm sling is all that is required. It is caused, generally, by direct violence.

Humerus

Unless grossly displaced or compound, treat with a collar-and-cuff or broad arm sling. This does not apply to supracondylar fractures (see **Elbow**, below). Different authorities recommend a variety of plasters for fractures of the humeral shaft: verify local preferences.

Elbow

Displaced fractures and dislocations (q.v.) about the elbow need expert handling from the start. This applies especially to fractures involving the epicondyles in children. Comparison views of the two elbows are useful in children, with their complicated epiphyses; what appears to be a minor flake fracture from the lateral humeral condyle actually represents a substantial injury, with separation of a large fragment, including the entire articular surface of the capitulum, needing accurate reduction. Always check the *radial pulse* and hand movements immediately, and keep checking.

It is very easy to miss fractures of the radial head or neck when looking at X-rays. Look at every radial head with this specifically in mind if there is local tenderness of the elbow; if there is strong clinical suspicion of a fracture but the X-ray is normal, treat with a sling and review and

X-ray again in about 12 days time, when any fracture should be visible.

Myositis ossificans is relatively common after elbow injuries, especially in children, and passive movements, including physiotherapy, should therefore be avoided.

Radius and ulna

These are difficult and very important to deal with well. In my opinion, they should be treated by an orthopaedic surgeon from the start. Refer immediately.

Colles' fracture

A very common fracture, particularly in elderly osteoporotic women. The fracture site is the distal radius and the distal fragment is displaced dorsally, angulated dorsally and displaced radially. It is also pulled proximally. The ulnar styloid may or may not be fractured. Dinner-fork deformity is usual; tenderness at the fracture site is invariable. X-ray confirms the diagnosis.

The initial decision is whether or not the fracture requires reduction and the principal factors involved are the age of the patient, whether his dominant hand is involved, his occupation and his interests, as well as the degree of displacement. A 30-year-old pianist will require more accurate reduction than an 85-year-old woman.

The most important angle is that between the shaft of the radius and its distal cup. This angle should normally be about 10° ventrally. In general, an angle of 0° is just about acceptable but would certainly not be accepted by a young patient (see Fig. 4a). An angle of −5° might be satisfactory in an old person with few requirements. Each case must be considered on its merits: nowhere else is this more true.

If reduction is not required, a backslab plaster of Paris is applied and the arm put into a broad arm sling. Give analgesia. The plaster is checked next day and completed (or changed for a complete plaster) in three or four days, when the swelling has resolved. A check X-ray is taken at ten days to ensure the satisfactory position is maintained.

If reduction is necessary, there is the choice of general anaesthesia or a Bier's block (see **Anaesthesia, local and regional**). Personally, all else being equal, I prefer the latter, which I have always found a safe and satisfactory (to myself and my patients) technique if performed correctly. The great advantages of a Bier's block are that it can be performed as soon as is convenient for the staff and the patient can go home within a few minutes of completion of the reduction.

Whichever method of anaesthesia is employed, the first step in reduction is to distract the two fragments: it is surprising how often attempts are made to push one piece of bone through another (see Fig. 4b). Gently pull the two fragments apart for two minutes or so: the surgeon pulls on the hand while an assistant provides counter-traction at the elbow. Following this distraction, it is advisable to increase the deformity slightly (extension at the fracture site) before reduction (flexion at the fracture site). Generally, the greater the initial displacement, the easier it is to obtain a good reduction.

The surgeon having satisfied himself with the reduction, comparing the two wrists by palpation, a backslab plaster is applied with the wrist in moderate flexion and moderate ulnar deviation (see Fig. 4c). The forearm is in pronation during reduction and plastering. A check X-ray is taken, to confirm satisfactory reduction. If unsatisfactory, have another attempt while the patient (or his wrist) is still anaesthetized. It follows that a patient having a general anaesthetic should be kept unconscious until the post-reduction films have been approved by the surgeon: ensure the anaesthetist knows this.

Send the patient home with a broad arm sling, adequate analgesia, plaster instructions (see **Plaster of Paris**) and an appointment to be seen next day.

The plaster is checked next day and completed in 4 days or so, when the swelling has subsided. A check X-ray is taken at about 10 days; slippage is very unlikely after this time, whereas if it has already occurred the fracture is still shiftable and re-reduction can be performed.

The plaster is removed at about 6 weeks and union is assessed both clinically and radiologically. A decision is

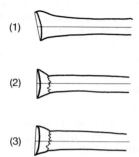

(a) 1. The normal angle is 10° ventrally, 2. 0° is just about acceptable, 3. −5° is seldom acceptable.

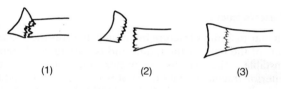

(b) 1 must be converted to 3 via 2; it cannot go directly from 1 to 3.

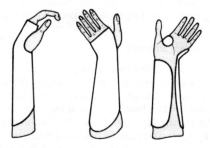

(c) The backslab holds the wrist in moderate flexion and moderate ulnar deviation.

Fig. 4

made whether physiotherapy is needed and a supporting bandage is provided for another 2 weeks or so.

Clearly function of the wrist is the most important aspect of the final result but most people understandably require a reasonably acceptable cosmetic result also.

Smith's fracture

The reverse of Colles' fracture, i.e. fracture of the distal end of the radius with anterior displacement of the distal fragment. This can be difficult to reduce and it is important to reduce it fully to avoid disability afterwards. Don't forget that it requires an above-elbow plaster of Paris with the forearm in full supination to avoid redisplacement. Admit overnight to ensure supervision of the circulation.

Barton's fracture

Similar to Smith's fracture but it only involves the anterior part of the base of the radius and is therefore inherently unstable. The carpus dislocates anteriorly with the anterior fragment (see Fig. 5). It is not difficult to reduce but requires to be put in full supination with extension of the wrist in an above-elbow plaster of Paris. Some surgeons prefer to do open reduction and internal fixation as a routine. It is not all that common and so worth discussing with an orthopaedic surgeon when it arises.

'Juvenile Colles' fracture'

This is not strictly a fracture but a posterior displacement of the radial epiphysis in a patient under the age of 20 years (but usually under 15). There is generally a dorsal flake of bone broken from the radial metaphysis. It can be difficult to manipulate satisfactorily. Prolonged traction followed by forced flexion of the wrist first and then very firm digital pressure over the dorsum of the epiphysis is required. A below-elbow plaster of Paris is used, with the forearm in strongly applied pronation. This is a stable fracture after full reduction.

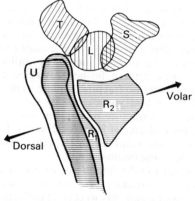

Fig. 5. Barton's fracture/dislocation of the wrist. U, ulna; R_1, shaft of radius; R_2, anterior distal fragment; T, triquetral; L, lunate; S, scaphoid.

Carpal fractures

Scaphoid fractures are the commonest and most important because of the risk of non-union or avascular necrosis of the proximal fragment when the fracture is at the waist. Ask the radiographer for 'scaphoid views' if there is tenderness in the scaphoid area, including in the anatomical snuff box. If there is a fracture, apply a scaphoid plaster of Paris (thumb opposed to the middle finger and proximal phalanx included), and refer the patient to fracture clinic. But fractures of the scaphoid do not always show up immediately on X-ray and so, if no fracture is seen on X-ray but local clinical signs are convincing, apply a scaphoid plaster of Paris, X-ray again, out of plaster, after 2 weeks (by which stage a fracture will almost certainly be visible), and act accordingly; review the patient again after a further 2 weeks, even if the second X-ray shows no fracture; explain to the patient on the day of injury that you cannot be sure at that stage whether there is a fracture or not, but you have to play safe and apply a plaster of Paris for 2 weeks. Fractures of the tubercle of the scaphoid rarely cause problems and require symptomatic treatment only.

Be sure never to miss fracture-dislocations such as the trans-scaphoid perilunate fracture-dislocation. It is agonizingly painful and easy to correct early; not so later.

After a few years in an accident department there will be no carpal bone you have not seen fractured. They usually require symptomatic treatment with plaster of Paris for 3 or 4 weeks. Subsequent arthritic complications may require arthrodesis or removal of a markedly deformed carpal bone. Lunates usually, but not always, dislocate before they break.

■ Fractures, hand

It is rare for these to need extensive treatment or even reduction. Multiple fractures of metacarpals or other serious hand injuries need admission for specialist care. Crush injury produces disorganization of hand function and is always a major problem which requires expert assessment and care. *Serious hand injury is an emergency and must always be treated as such.* When you are in doubt about the adequacy of simple support for a hand fracture, seek advice from your consultant or an orthopaedic or plastic surgeon. Every A & E department should provide full facilities for emergency treatment of major or multiple hand injuries. They are of unparalleled importance to the patient, and the possibilities of salvage at primary operation are endless. They do, however, need experience, time, and the maximum of effort if good results are to be achieved. Strive to ensure that every such patient has the opportunity of the best possible care. If your own hospital does not offer an adequate hand service, for the patient's sake refer him to another hospital that does. Too much depends on primary care for risks to be taken. Elevation is always mandatory from the start; early mobilization is important.

Special fractures of the hand

Bennett's fracture-dislocation of the thumb   Anatomical reduction is essential. This may be stable in an abduction plaster with a small felt pad over the base of the first metacarpal. If not, it needs internal fixation with a K-wire or screw (see Fig. 6).

Shaft of first metacarpal   An unstable fracture which may be stabilized in an abduction plaster, but needs an intramedullary K-wire if not.

Second to fifth metacarpal shafts   Unstable fractures may need internal fixation. Stable fractures without gross displacement need neighbour-strapping of the relevant fingers and a metacarpal pad for about 3 weeks and do well.

Fig. 4 ...

...

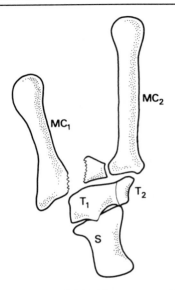

Fig. 6. Bennett's fracture/dislocation: an unstable injury. T_1, trapezium; T_2, trapezoid; S, scaphoid; MC_1 and MC_2, first and second metacarpals.

'Punch' fracture of fifth metacarpal neck Reduction makes this fracture unstable and should not be attempted. Treat it by neighbour-strapping the 2 medial fingers for 3 weeks. The deformity will be permanent but slight, and function will be normal.

Phalangeal fractures Splint with neighbour-strapping, which allows mobility but gives support. Some fractures are essentially unstable, notably oblique fractures involving the distal articular surface; these can sometimes be stabilized with a small K-wire.

When you see a patient with a fracture of a long bone in the hand (especially a proximal phalanx), ensure you see him make a fist; rotational deformity may be obvious in

flexion but undetected in extension. Early reduction is needed to prevent permanent deformity; internal fixation may be necessary.

Button-hole fracture of the terminal phalanx, in which the metaphyseal fragment is extruded and caught superficial to the nail fold, has to be carefully 'shoe-horned' in and under the nail fold and put in an extension splint.

Abduction fracture of the proximal phalanx of the little finger in children must always be reduced before neighbour-strapping. This is generally a juxta-epiphyseal greenstick fracture of the metaphysis of the proximal phalanx. If treated wrongly it leads to an unsightly and inconvenient deformity.

Mallet finger is often associated with a marginal fracture of the base of the terminal phalanx. The standard, plastic, mallet-finger splint can give approximately 85% success rate if applied early and meticulously supervised; about 6 weeks incessant support are needed.

The earliest mobilization of these fractures is vital. Various types of internal and external splintage are used to achieve this and expert advice should always be sought.

See also **Hand infections and injuries**

Fractures, lower limb

Femur, neck

Tie the feet together as first aid if pain is severe.

Femur, shaft

Apply Thomas's splint with adhesive traction for first aid and before radiography. Give intravenous analgesia before moving the patient. Femoral nerve block (see **Anaesthesia, local and regional**) should always be used before splintage.

Knee (above and below)

These are difficult fractures and need admission. The X-ray appearances of fractures of the tibial plateau can be difficult to interpret, particularly with depressed fractures, in which a fracture line as such can be virtually invisible; consequently these fractures are missed with depressing frequency. They are well described in standard texts. See **Bibliography**.

Patella

If there is separation or comminution, admit. Splint in extension for first aid. 'Toffee in paper' fracture needs a plaster of Paris cylinder. Do not be caught out by congenital bipartite patella, which is often (but not always) bilateral.

Tibia and fibula (shafts)

An unstable fracture needing expert mending; a foam trough is better than an inflatable splint for first aid support and radiography. Manipulation and an above-knee plaster of Paris are needed after orthopaedic consultation. Better reduction with less risk of angulation is achieved by using the vertical position with the knee flexed over the end of the trolley: the plaster should then be applied in 3 parts, first the leg while traction on the heel is maintained, then the foot, then the above-knee portion. Compound fractures need careful wound toilet and closure as well as full antibiotic cover and tetanus protection before manipulation and plastering. Remember that such fractures represent blood loss of between one and two units. Admit.

Ankle

Pott's All degrees of Pott's fracture require plaster of Paris but there is wide divergence of opinion about when internal fixation should be used. You will have to find out what the relevant orthopaedic surgeon prefers and act accordingly.

Fibular   Below the inferior tibio-fibular joint, plaster of Paris is required; above the inferior tibio-fibular joint (undisplaced), double Tubigrip is satisfactory, or plaster of Paris if pain is persistent. If there is diastasis at the inferior tibio-fibular joint, internal fixation may be required. Look for a fracture at the fibular neck in cases of inferior tibio-fibular diastasis: it is an indicator of Maisonneuve fracture; in this type the interosseous membrane itself may split, so that the two bones open apart like a pair of tongs; this is very much an orthopaedic problem, needing open reduction and internal fixation; cf. **Ankle**, ruptured ligaments of the.

Unstable ankle fractures and ligamentous injuries   Except for unstable fractures of the malleoli, which need internal fixation, ligamentous injuries must always be demonstrated radiographically by means of stressed inversion/eversion X-rays under general anaesthesia. Rupture of the medial ligament of the ankle needs operative repair, and of the lateral ligament plaster of Paris in a slightly everted and extended position of the ankle joint for six weeks (cf. **Ankle**). Some repair both, others repair neither. Rational investigation of the efficacy of these contradictory approaches seems to be needed.

Foot

Calcaneus   This is common after jumping. There is tenderness on lateral compression; it is a painful and disabling injury. X-ray appearances can be misleading, particularly with compression fractures, because (as with depressed fractures of the tibial plateau) a fracture line as such may not be visible; but the upper surface of the calcaneus is distinctly flattened, so that the line of the subtalar joint may form almost a straight line with the upper surface of the tuberosity; this angle is normally about 40°. Severely swollen injuries benefit from high elevation. Tubigrip and crutches are needed, with ultrasound for pain. Some surgeons reduce all flattened fractures; others reduce none of them. Some recommend primary subtalar fusion for bad calcaneal fractures.

Transmitted violence may produce associated fractures of the tibial plateau, dorso-lumbar spine, and odontoid peg. If severe, admit for elevation and review.

Talus and other tarsal bones   These fractures are comparatively rare. Local tenderness is diagnostic. Specify the site of local signs to the radiographer and radiologist. Orthopaedic advice is needed in cases of fracture, especially of the talus and navicular.

Metatarsals   These are common fractures, especially the base of the fifth metatarsal in acute inversion injuries: this only needs support except for the rare cases of gross displacement. Other metatarsal shafts (especially stress fractures of the second or third metatarsals, of which the only radiological sign may be callus formation) need only support and rest, unless they are much displaced. Varieties of transverse tarsal fractures and tarsal crush injuries occur rarely and need specialist assessment from the beginning. Distal and mid-tarsal fracture-dislocations are very destructive injuries; painstaking realignment and fixation are specialist problems.

Phalanges   These fractures are very common in industrial and domestic accidents and are usually satisfactorily treated by neighbour-strapping. In crush injuries with avulsion of nails or burst injuries, don't forget that these fractures are compound and need full antibiotic and tetanus protection. Exploration and reconstruction may be required as in crushed fingers (see **Hand infections and injuries**).

Stress fractures

For example, fracture of the shaft of the second metatarsal. There is gradual onset of pain with no early X-ray changes and the fracture may not be spotted until the excess callus of an unstable fracture is visible. Immobilization for 6 weeks may be needed. Stress fractures can also occur in an athlete's tibia.

■ Gas gangrene

Gas gangrene is especially likely to develop in deep, dirty, and contused wounds. It should be avoided by meticulous debridement of the wound, excision of all non-viable tissue, and a prophylactic intramuscular injection of Triplopen (see **Antibiotics**).

■ Gastro-intestinal emergencies

Briefly reviewed as a far-from-complete *aide-mémoire*:

Gastro-intestinal haemorrhages

- **Oesophageal varices**
- **Mallory–Weiss syndrome** (bleeding after vomiting)
- **Bleeding peptic ulcers**
- **Haemangiomata**
- **Meckel's diverticulum** (containing ectopic gastric mucosa)
- **Carcinoma** of the rectum more commonly than of the colon

See **Collapse and coma; Haematological emergencies**

Obstructive syndromes

- **Hypertrophic pyloric stenosis in infants**   Usually a male first-born, 3–8 weeks old, with projectile vomiting and a palpable tumour while feeding. It can occur in females and siblings.
- **Volvulus of loops of small intestine** round or through adhesions, Meckel's diverticulum, or what not.
- **Strangulated   herniae**   Umbilical,   inguinal, femoral, and obturator.
- **Various neonatal atresias**
- **Intussusception**   Intermittent vomiting and colic in bonny boys, 6–9 months old. A palpable tumour is far from universal.

- **Gall stone ileus**
- **Faecal impaction** in elderly, debilitated patients presents from time to time with pelvic pain and pseudo-diarrhoea. Manual removal is required.
- **Neoplastic disease**

Miscellaneous

- **Appendicitis**
- **Gall bladder disease**
- **Pancreatitis**
- **Diverticulitis**
- **Crohn's disease**
- **Acute rectal prolapse** in infants needs gentle manipulative reduction, strapping of the buttocks, and admission; it may be due to cystic fibrosis.
- **Abdominal trauma** is a separate subject and is dealt with under **Abdominal injuries** (q.v.).
- **Food poisoning** (q.v.).

■ General practitioners

Friendly and close collaboration with local General Practitioners is one of the foundation stones of successful management of an accident unit.

If the General Practitioners provide a conscientious service to their patients (which in my experience they do magnificently) the unit can get on with treating accidents and emergencies. As a *quid pro quo* the unit should be ready at all times to help with urgent diagnostic conundrums and can often provide an invaluable service in regular sessions for non-urgent minor surgery. Urgent minor surgery is our responsibility anyhow.

■ Gout and pseudo-gout

Gout is a common cause of acute arthrosis (not only in the first metatarsophalangeal joint) in adults of all ages, and rarely in children. It often presents as traumatic in origin; sometimes a history of minor trauma is genuine but often it has been added by the patient as a rationalization of his pain and does not stand up to questioning. It is identified by the following signs:

- Pain in the joint unrelieved by rest
- Local redness, tenderness, and swelling, with heat, but without fever
- Absence of a history of trauma proportionate to the symptoms
- Raised serum uric acid (inconstant and unreliable)
- Tophi in the pinnae
- Uric acid crystals on joint aspiration

X-ray in acute gout shows only soft tissue swelling; in chronic gout, there are punched-out lesions in the juxta-articular bone. The initial treatment consists of colchicine or naproxen: a response within 48 hours is characteristic. Allopurinol is prophylactic only and should not be given in the acute attack; whether any further treatment beyond the immediate one is required is a matter for a physician to decide.

Calcium pyrophosphate crystal deposition (pseudo-gout) is diagnosed in acute cases by identification of the crystals after joint aspiration, and in chronic cases by fluffy calcification in periarticular soft tissues. It is a good deal less responsive to all forms of treatment than the genuine variety, but a non-steroidal anti-inflammatory drug may help.

■ Grafts, skin

In accident work there are four types of skin graft which may be useful:

Pinch grafts

For small finger repairs (excluding fingertip ablations which are better dealt with by V–Y plasty or volar flaps: see **Hand infections and injuries**). These grafts are done by raising a weal on the hairless skin of the forearm and slicing off the bleb with a scalpel blade. They are transferred to the denuded area after careful cleaning and debridement, fixed with four 6/0 monofilament stitches, flattened, covered with a single layer of chlorhexidine tulle and a firm pressure bandage, and left in place for 5 days in a sling for elevation. Cover the donor area with chlorhexidine tulle. After 5 days the grafts are inspected *very carefully* and lightly dressed as the situation demands. Once well 'taken' the graft should be kept well greased.

Split skin grafts

Can readily be taken from the donor area under local anaesthesia. These grafts are useful for *backs* of hands and feet with extensive skin deficit. With experience small Thiersch grafts can be cut with a scalpel, but Silver's graft knife is simpler. They should be handled very carefully, stitched in place with 6/0 monofilament sutures and punctured with a scalpel after fixation so as to prevent formation of haematoma or seroma.

A firm dressing for 5 days is essential. Chlorhexidine tulle (Bactigras) is the best first layer to avoid sticking.

Pedicle grafts

Useful for full thickness skin loss from fingers, but best left to the experts as in-patient treatment is necessary. Small pedicle grafts for fingers do not require Thiersch grafting to the donor area as primary suture will generally close the deficiency.

Wolfe (full thickness) grafts

Not as reliable as the above but may be attempted when a patient brings in the skin he has lost. The autograft should be defatted completely and with care, and the graft thoroughly washed first in saline and then in cetrimide (0.5% solution). It needs to be fixed with numerous fine peripheral stitches and pierced to avoid formation of haematoma. A pad and bandage provide compression and the whole should be left alone for 5 days at least. Oral antibiotics and elevation of the limb are necessary.

■ Gunshot wounds

In general, gunshot wounds with major damage occur in young people and need early blood volume replacement.

Airgun

Remove subcutaneous pellets and leave deeper ones unless they are near vital structures, e.g. in the wrist. Pellets land in the orbit surprisingly commonly and should be referred for an ophthalmic opinion urgently.

.22 rifle

The same rules apply, with the proviso that the bullet must be carefully localized by X-ray. Abdominal wounds need to be regarded with extreme suspicion, as visceral perforations can occur with a minimum of initial symptoms and signs, and no demonstrable track.

.410 shotgun

Dangerous only at close range (a few feet). Although the explosive charge is small the muzzle velocity is high enough to do considerable damage. For instance, of two injuries due to stumbling when holding a loaded .410, one necessitated resection of the right lobe of the liver after ligature of the right hepatic artery, and the other resulted in death due to multiple perforations of the aortic bifurcation with massive haematoperitoneum.

Twelve-bore shotgun

A very much more powerful gun which can produce extensive damage at a range of several yards. Suicidal shooting through the mouth is immensely destructive. Stray pellets are an occasional finding in routine X-rays of rural patients and require no action. The sawn-off shotgun is a familiar cause of destructive injuries at close range owing to the rapid spread of the charge. The injuries require definitive surgical treatment according to general anatomical and surgical principles. They are difficult cases to deal with owing to the wide extent of tissue damage and skin destruction. Urgent resuscitation and blood transfusion are generally required.

Military missile systems
(e.g. Armalite and other high velocity rifles)

These have their own characteristics and are dealt with in specialist literature (see **Bibliography**).

Explosive bullets

An increasing menace for surgeons and pathologists following criminal assaults (Knight, B. (1982). Explosive bullets: a new hazard for doctors. *British Medical Journal*, **284**, 768–9).

Gunshot and bomb blast injuries are particularly frequent in Northern Ireland (Roy, D. (1982). Gunshot and bomb blast injuries: a review of experience in Belfast. *Journal of the Royal Society of Medicine*, **75**, 542–5).

■ Gynaecological emergencies

- **Abortion** (q.v.)
- **Ectopic pregnancy** There is low abdominal pain and amenorrhoea; bleeding is not always present.
- **Endometriosis** Can present as acute pelvic pain; tender ovarian cysts may be present; the symptoms are often related to menstruation.
- **Ovarian cysts** Bleeding into or torsion of.
- **Salpingitis** This is acutely painful and tender and the patient is febrile; vaginal discharge is not always present.
- **Vulvovaginitis** Can have a very acute onset and present at night or weekends; warm bicarbonate bathing and/or douching is a good first aid measure.
- **Trichomonal and candidal infections** Should be investigated with high vaginal swabs for culture and sensitivity; treatment with oral metronidazole or antifungal pessaries can be initiated; predisposing causes (diabetes, poor hygiene, malnutrition, and debility) should be excluded; return the patient to the care of the General Practitioner.

Cf. **Obstetric emergencies; Venereal disease**

■ Haematological emergencies

Examples of those presenting in A & E departments from time to time include the following:

Abnormal bleeding

1 *Congenital*
   Haemophilia
   Christmas disease
   von Willebrand's disease
2 *Iatrogenic*
   Warfarin
   Heparin
   Dindevan
3 *Thrombocytopenia*
   Idiopathic
   Secondary (e.g. to leukaemia)

Hereditary haemoglobinopathies

Sickle cell disease
Thalassaemia

These patients should be discussed with a haematologist (or a physician) at the earliest opportunity: they are often known already. Patients with haemophilia or Christmas disease should carry cards and are usually registered at one of the haemophilia centres and the finer details of their management should be left to the experts. A telephone call to a doctor at the haemophilia centre will often yield useful advice and prevent disastrous therapeutic errors. These patients are normally well informed as to whether or not specific treatment (cryoprecipitate or whatever) is required.

The management of an acute haemarthrosis or a suspected (by the patient) haemarthrosis in a haemophiliac should be undertaken only after detailed consultation with a haematologist and an orthopaedic surgeon. Joint aspiration can usually be avoided if early treatment is given.

If a patient with haemophilia (or Christmas disease) has sustained an injury, take a specimen of blood in a prothrombin bottle for factor VIII (or IX) level, and then give appropriate clotting factor replacement therapy. This should, of course, be done in consultation with a haematologist.

In cases of bleeding in patients receiving oral anticoagulants, the prothrombin time should be carried out as an urgent investigation.

In Negro patients presenting with bone pain, an emergency test for sickle cell haemoglobin should be performed.

But at the end of the day (and at the beginning), the management of these patients is the responsibility of the haematologist, not the casualty officer.

■ Hand infections and injuries

Cf. **Fractures, hand; Tendon repairs, hand; Wrist and hand amputations**

You *must* know how to examine an injured or infected hand. If you examine *all the movements* of all the fingers, and the thumb, and the wrist, and *sensation throughout* the hand, you won't miss much.

Test flexor digitorum profundus to each finger by nolding the proximal interphalangeal joint in extension and ensure the patient can actively flex the distal interphalangeal joint. Test flexor digitorum superficialis to each finger by holding the other three fingers in extension and ensure the patient can actively flex the proximal interphalangeal joint. You must also test flexion at the metacarpophalangeal joints, and extension, abduction and adduction of each of the fingers. Don't forget the movements of the thumb (flexion, extension, abduction, adduction, and opposition). Partial division of a tendon may subsequently become complete: always test very carefully, record what you find, and refer upwards if you feel unsure.

The finer details of the anatomy of the hand can be found in textbooks devoted to the hand (see **Bibliography**).

How much you are able to do in the way of surgery depends on:

- The facilities available to you, including use of an operating theatre and the availability of in-patient beds
- The staff available to you: no hand surgery is possible without adequate assistance
- The time available to you
- Your expertise

There are a number of excellent books on the subject. Consult them if you intend to progress beyond the basics, as given here. See **Bibliography**. Always seek advice if you feel unsure: wrong treatment at the onset can have disastrous consequences.

Dressings to fingers should be kept to a minimum and done without if possible. Early movement takes precedence always. An ugly finger that moves is better than a beautiful finger that doesn't. Elevation is vital. Rehabilitation and intensive physiotherapy and occupational therapy are often needed.

Crushed terminal phalanx

If there is fragmentation of the bone with displacement and soft tissue injury, exploration under digital nerve block is essential. Detached fragments should be removed and careful suture performed. Neglect of this can lead to sequestration of fragments and long-delayed recovery. Intramuscular antibiotic is advisable. Tetanus protection is required. Give a 5-day course of oral antibiotic (e.g. Augmentin) after all compound injuries.

Subungual haematoma

See **Nails, digital**

Burst finger

A common industrial accident. The prognosis is often bad in view of the vascular damage and the poor viability of the tissues. Do the minimum of repairs: sling, high dose antibiotics. Refer to specialist care if required. Primary closure may be essential to obtain skin cover.

Lacerations

Provided nerve and tendon damage is absent and the blood supply is good, suture carefully with monofilament nylon or polypropylene, which gives the best scars; the finer the better provided the grade is appropriate to the wound. In children a lot can be done with adhesive skin-closure strips, because the skin is soft; this is both kinder and more effective, when circumstances permit.

Digital nerve repair is generally accepted as a primary procedure more likely to give quicker and more effective recovery of sensation than not. It should be done by an expert.

Amputated finger tips

Partial thickness or full thickness without loss of pulp (i.e. some dermal remnants): allow to epithelialize.

Full thickness with pulp loss or exposure of terminal phalanx: if you can do it a V–Y plasty is best; if not, refer for specialist attention.

V–Y plasty

The purpose of this simple and elegant operation is to provide two symmetrical sliding pedicle grafts from the sides of the finger which can be brought up to unite over the denuded fingertip (see Fig. 7). It provides skin cover of the right type, carrying its own blood and nerve supply (Kutler, W. (1947). A new method for finger tip amputation. *Journal of the American Medical Association*, **133**, 29–30). A similar V–Y advancement of volar skin can be used to attach oblique sliding grafts of the volar pulp of a finger or thumb. This technique provides cosmetically well in younger patients with defects and has the 'advantage' of leaving a flat insertion line. For Tranquilli-Leali's technique, see Barron, J. N. and Emmett, A. J. J. (1965). *Br. J. Plast. Surg.* **18**, 51. Reproduced from the experimental figure up with a muscular skin flap. *Acta orthop. Scand.* and *Joint Surgery*.

Fig. 8. (a) and (b)... defect oblique and is no less than 1.5 cm at its deepest. (c)... over the bottom as to make sure the deep as the new skin...including in the top part reattachment flap will pull...is parallel with transferred ellipses, and advances...

used to repair oblique ablations of the whole pulp of a finger or thumb; it is easier to perform and works well in younger patients with soft skins, but has the disadvantage of leaving a volar scar (see Fig. 8) (Atasoy, E., Ioakimidis, E., Kasdan, M. L., Kutz, J. E. and Kleinert, H. E. (1970). Reconstruction of the amputated finger tip with a triangular volar flap. *Journal of Bone and Joint Surgery* [American edition], **52A**, 921–6).

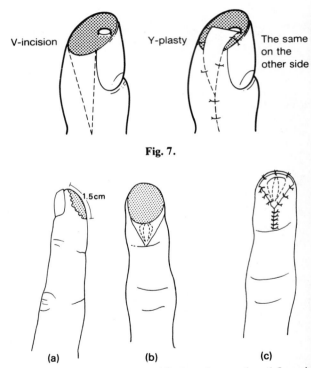

Fig. 7.

Fig. 8. (a) Pulp amputation: oblique and more than 1.5 cm in length; (b) the V-incision: the broken lines represents the deep neuro-vascular pedicles; (c) the V-shaped advancement flap with pedicle, sutured in position with interrupted stitches, and Y-closure.

Traumatic amputations

These require careful terminalization of the remaining phalanges. Volar flaps to cover the finger end should be used whenever possible, even at the cost of small additional shortening, because in the result they are superior to terminal scars or Wolfe grafts.

Avulsion of fingers

This injury occurs in lathe and drill workers whose gloves, catching in the rotating component, are twisted rapidly with the fingers inside them. The avulsion is usually at the metacarpophalangeal joint and the tendons and nerves may be pulled out at considerable length. Refer to an expert.

Amputations

If a finger or thumb has been amputated in an accident replantation may be possible: refer to an expert immediately. If you think amputation may be necessary, refer upwards: the finer details of the various procedures available—and what is best for each particular patient—is for the experts to decide. Having decided that amputation is inescapable, the choice lies between length and function of the resulting digits. The most careful consideration of every aspect of the patient's interests and welfare must always be taken before embarking on such a disfiguring operation.

Collateral ligaments

These are injured in side-to-side wrenching accidents. Those of the interphalangeal joints of the fingers should generally be repaired; otherwise a troublesome instability remains.

A ruptured ulnar collateral ligament of the first metacarpophalangeal joint (gamekeeper's thumb) should always be repaired. Rupture is readily identified by firm radial deviation of the thumb whenever local pain

swelling, and tenderness suggest local injury. If it is not repaired, permanent, disabling instability, with loss of pinch, ensues. It needs early identification (with stress X-rays under local anaesthesia) and early repair. Always look for it when examining a 'sprained' thumb.

High pressure injection injuries

A grease-gun can exert pressures up to 10 000 lb/sq in, producing tissue necrosis and vascular coagulation; in addition grease may enter a tissue plane or tendon sheath and travel a long way. Such destructive injuries need wide exploration and opening to the extreme limits so as to allow profuse irrigation and debridement. Refer to an expert. Delayed amputation may be required but it should not be delayed too long; as soon as the destruction of the skin circulation of (for instance) a digit is established, amputation should be carried out to shorten the time of disability and allow an early return to work.

Blackthorn injuries

These are common and very painful in hedgers. They always need careful exploration as the tiniest residue of blackthorn bark generally produces a painful aseptic abscess. The thorn is so tough and the hedger's blows so energetic that joints and articular cartilage are not uncommonly transfixed. Removal produces rapid relief of pain and swelling.

Infections

Paronychia (whitlow), pulp infection, and other deep infections of the fingers can be perfectly well dealt with under digital nerve block provided the local anaesthetic is injected into healthy tissue and concurrent antibiotic given in adequate dosage. The secret of success is adequate exposure, exploration, and drainage.

Chronic paronychia (fungal or monilial with secondary bacterial overtones) can dawdle on for months with

painful episodes of secondary infection. Make a combined attack with local toilet of the nail-fold, oral antibiotics, and prolonged topical antifungal/monilial agents, e.g. 1% clotrimazole cream (Canesten). Oral systemically-acting fungicides help, e.g. griseofulvin 500 mg twice a day. Topical applications should be used for three weeks at least.

Palmar space infections and abscesses involving tendon sheaths require the fullest exploration, drainage, antibiotics, elevation, and aftercare. Refer to an expert.

Major infections need parenteral antibiotics 8-hourly for 24 hours or longer, as well as proper drainage.

■ Hay fever

Can be of such acute and severe onset as to constitute a genuine emergency. When there is a combination of conjunctival chemosis with upper respiratory congestion, and sometimes wheezing as well, it is necessary to give urgent relief.

This situation arises commonly at the height of the grass pollen season when contact has been close and intense (e.g. a sensitive child playing in long grass) and needs intravenous antihistamine, e.g. chlorpheniramine (Piriton) 10 mg, followed by steroid injection, e.g. intramuscular methylprednisolone (Depo-Medrone) 80 mg, if relief is inadequate.

Acute chemosis of the conjunctiva (so much more distressing to the observers than the patient) can be relieved by instillation of 1% adrenaline eye-drops (Eppy), one or two drops at a time, until a response is achieved.

Sodium cromoglycate eye-drops 2% (Opticrom) are useful for allergic conjunctivitis and sodium cromoglycate nasal drops 2% (Rynacrom) are recommended for severe nasal allergy.

All such cases should be referred to their own GP for consideration for a hyposensitization course.

■ Head injuries

The most crucial contribution to the recovery of severe head injuries that can be made in an accident unit is the immediate establishment of an airway and adequate oxygenation in all cases. This may involve cuffed endotracheal intubation on reception of the injured person, even laryngostomy (q.v.) in cases with severe mandibular or submandibular injuries who have laryngeal occlusion, and the provision of proper means of intravenous infusion.

The essence of the early management of head injuries is to detect deterioration as early as possible, and it follows that baseline observations should be performed as soon as possible, and repeated frequently thereafter. These include pulse, blood pressure, temperature, respiratory rate, pupil size and reaction, limb movement and power in all four limbs, examination of the central nervous system, and, most important of all, the conscious level. The latter is best measured by use of the Glasgow Coma Scale (Teasdale, G. and Jennett, B. (1974). Assessment of coma and impaired consciousness. *Lancet*, **ii**, 81–4), which combines the two essential qualities of sensitivity and lack of ambiguity.

The casualty officer dealing with a patient who has sustained a head injury has 3 basic questions to answer:

1　Is a skull X-ray necessary?
2　Is admission necessary?
3　Is consultation with a neurosurgeon necessary?

There are no general answers to any of these questions and each case must be taken on its merits. Eminent surgeons have produced guidelines (A group of neurosurgeons (1984). Guidelines for initial management after head injury in adults. *British Medical Journal*, **288**, 983–5), which are of great value, but clinical judgement is always necessary.

Skull X-ray is necessary after recent head injury if there is

- Loss of consciousness or amnesia at any time
- Neurological symptoms or signs
- Cerebrospinal fluid or blood from the nose or ear
- Suspected penetrating injury
- Scalp bruising or swelling

Admission is necessary if there is:

- Confusion or any other depression of the level of consciousness at the time of examination
- Skull fracture
- Neurological symptoms or signs
- Difficulty in assessing the patient—for example, alcohol, epilepsy, or other medical condition (e.g. haemophilia); also young children
- Lack of a responsible adult to supervise the patient; other social problems
- Vomiting

Note: Brief amnesia after trauma with full recovery is not sufficient indication for admission. In the absence of witnesses amnesia is the significant indication of concussion. Relatives or friends of patients sent home should receive written advice about changes that would require the patient to be returned urgently to hospital. A suggested form is as follows:

Instructions following a minor head injury
You should return to the hospital or contact your own doctor if the following symptoms occur:
> *Severe headache*
> *Vomiting*
> *Drowsiness*
> *Dizziness*
> *Eye trouble*

or if you become concerned about the condition of the patient.

Consultation with a neurosurgeon (and access to computerized axial tomography) is necessary if there is:

- Fractured skull with any of the following: confusion or impairment of consciousness, one or more epileptic fits, or any other neurological symptoms or signs
- Coma continuing after resuscitation—even if there is no skull fracture
- Deterioration in the level of consciousness

- Confusion or impaired remembrance of occurrences preceding the injury even if there is no overt trauma.
- Depressed fracture of the skull.
- Suspected fracture of the base of the skull (e.g. bruising round the eyes or round the ears, blood or ... appearing from the nose and ears, etc.)
- ... haemorrhage ... to the ... by ambulance ...

If patients are to be transferred to another hospital, the following are necessary:

- They should be nursed on their ...
- Initial wound ... and, for extra-cranial injuries and ... controlled ... to prevent shock. In shock, blood and ... replacement and ... and ...
- ... conscious patients ... ... to the hospital to which they are to be transferred by ... (usually ambulance) and communication with the ...
- Send if necessary X-ray films.

...

See also ...

- Confusion or other neurological disturbances persisting for more than 8 hours, even if there is no skull fracture
- Depressed fracture of the skull vault
- Suspected fracture of the base of the skull (cerebrospinal fluid rhinorrhoea or otorrhoea, bilateral orbital haematoma, mastoid haematoma, or evidence of a penetrating type of injury such as a spike or gunshot).

If patients are to be transferred to another hospital, the following are necessary:

- They should be referred urgently
- Initial resuscitation for extracranial injuries and complications must be completed (e.g. for shock, blood loss, compromised ventilation), and first aid for limb fractures
- Ensure precautions to reduce risks *en route* to the neurological unit (adequately equipped ambulance and a trained doctor or nurse as escort)
- Send all notes and X-ray films

Progressive changes occurring in the first few hours can give an urgent indication for specialist intervention, possibly to relieve increasing intracranial pressure by means of burr-holes; but this is unusual. Early deterioration is generally due to diffuse cerebral changes that are not amenable to surgery. This, however, is not the place to give detailed advice, and reference should be made to standard works on head injuries (see **Bibliography**).

There is dispute about the use of steroids where brain damage is severe, but current feeling is that they should be avoided. Osmotic diuretics (e.g. mannitol 25%) should only be given on the direct instruction of a neurosurgeon; their effectiveness is not in dispute but is of a 'once only' kind and cannot be repeated.

See also **Neurological emergencies** and **Antibiotics**

■ Hip syndrome, painful

This condition, common in children, can sometimes be regarded as a simple traumatic synovitis. It is characterized by a painful limp and relieved by not bearing weight. The leading physical sign is limitation of abduction and external rotation of the femur. It is often clearly unimportant, but in cases occurring between the ages of 4 and 9 years it should be regarded as a possible presentation of Perthes' disease. Occurring at puberty it may be due to slipped upper femoral epiphysis. In the first age group the hips should be X-rayed one month after the onset, if symptoms persist (with genital screening); exposure to X-rays is contra-indicated at the onset. In the second age group early X-ray is important. *Painful hip syndrome is an orthopaedic problem and reference to an orthopaedic surgeon is always necessary.* Treatment consists in encouraging rest and non-weightbearing until the pain and limp have subsided. If there is fever don't forget that osteomyelitis or septic arthritis are still possibilities. A simple toxic arthritis (e.g. concurrent with acute tonsillitis) explains some cases.

■ Hyperthermia and heat-stroke

Due to derangement of thermoregulation caused by salt and water depletion; it may be made worse by infective pyrexia at the same time. It is commoner in children in hot weather and still more so in those with fibrocystic disease. The rectal temperature may reach 43–45 °C. Rapid cooling by use of sheets soaked in cold water and dried by an electric fan should be continued till the rectal temperature falls to 39 °C. Set up an intravenous infusion of saline. Admit to the intensive care unit. If the temperature remains above 43 °C for long, irreversible brain damage ensues. Too rapid cooling can lead to peripheral shutdown and consequently to a sudden rise of core temperature. Tepid bathing and continuous rectal temperature recording is probably the most effective regime.

Heat will evaporate, so give oxygen by face mask, intravenously, by the cannula that are used for tissue, intravenous calcium gluconate 10%, with ...l or ...by infusion if needed saline.

A similar condition (malignant hyperpyrexia) can follow anaesthesia with halothane and other anaesthetic agents. This is associated with ...al to rectal dominant predisposition. Treat adrenaline, a ...large sodium ... might prove ...is not been ... at what the nearest to the nearest to therapy unit.

Hypothermia

This is common after drowning, ... later winter, lying drunk in clothes of some kind, or in elderly falling with a fractured neck of femur and not seen found till next day in the apartment, in severity ...mated by ...of a rectal temperature, with a ... for reading thermometer, and are ... below $35\,^\circ C$ ... to be regarded as a danger if ... is diminished. On ... take venous blood for ... 2 mmol/l, and full blood count. When the body temperature is below $30\,^\circ C$ are ... the treatment by ... ... be supplemented by saline infusion heated in the warming ... $30\,^\circ C$. When shivering hypotension have met you are nursing ... give, and the ... of temperature which is most be ... by external ... warming, which can be considered ... the ... 4-10 mg, intravenous ...il. Admit ... within ... care of an supportive ... ... or electrical conversion ... ... with a thermal probe in the rectum make management of cases ... much ...

Complications ... main also ... minute, acute pulmonary ... and hypotension ... develops. Left block, sinus bradycardia, and ... are prolonged ... are dealt with on their merits ... ...right to be ... predisposes to cardiac arrest, ...

First aid measures include oxygen by face mask, intravenous hydrocortisone 100 mg and, for rigors, intravenous calcium gluconate 10%: 5–10 ml or by infusion in normal saline.

A similar condition (**malignant hyperpyrexia**) can follow anaesthesia with halothane and other anaesthetic agents. This is associated with an autosomal dominant predisposition. Treat with intravenous dantrolene sodium 1 mg/kg, repeated as required, and admit the patient to the intensive therapy unit.

■ Hypothermia

This is common after drowning in winter waters, lying drunk in a ditch all Saturday night, or solitary falling with a fractured neck or femur and not being found till next day by the neighbours. Its severity is estimated by taking a rectal temperature with a special low-reading thermometer, and any fall below 35 °C should be regarded as a demand for treatment. On reception take venous blood for biochemical profile and full blood count. When the body temperature is below 30 °C the routine treatment by enclosure in a foil envelope ('space-blanket') may need to be supplemented by saline infusion heated in the warming circuit to 39 °C. When shivering begins you know that you are making progress, and the return of consciousness is often heralded by extreme restlessness, which can be confidently controlled by a small dose of diazepam (5–10 mg intramuscularly). Admission under the care of an appropriate specialist is always required. An electrical continuous-reading thermometer with a thermal probe in the rectum makes management of such patients much easier.

Complications are ventricular fibrillation, acute pulmonary oedema, hypotensive shock, heart block, sinus bradycardia, and acute pancreatitis. These are dealt with on their merits. Too rapid re-warming predisposes to cardiac arrhythmias.

■ Impetigo

This is very common in children, often unrecognized, and generally inadequately treated. It is a staphylococcal infection, commonly around the mouth. Treat with topical chlortetracycline or, if the condition is severe with signs of toxaemia, flucloxacillin by mouth. Sodium hypochlorite can be used to remove crusts and exudate. Impetigo is often secondary to oral herpes simplex (see **Viruses**) and acyclovir may help if diagnosed early.

Cf. **Skin emergencies**

■ Infestation

Hardly accidental or very urgent in Britain, but a common incident which has to be coped with in people attending A & E units for various reasons.

In temperate climates fleas, lice, and mites are the front runners, ticks coming a poor fourth. Fortunately the first three are susceptible to gamma benzene hexachloride 1% in an appropriate form. If resistant strains develop, organophosphorus compounds like malathion 0.5% are effective but more toxic. Repeated applications may be required to fit the life cycle of the parasite. Ticks are usually solitary or nearly so and dealt with mechanically (see **Sheep tick**).

In tropical and subtropical regions the variety of infestations is much larger and includes numerous worms, tape worms (remember hydatid disease!), flukes, protozoa, and so on. Two diagnostic features common to the large majority and fever and eosinophilia.

Detailed description is out of place here but can be found in standard texts (see **Bibliography**). Advice about tropical infestations is available from:

The Liverpool School of Tropical Medicine
051-708-9393
The London (St. Pancras) Hospital for Tropical
Diseases 01-387-4411
East Birmingham Hospital 021-772-4311

■ Injuries, minor

Pretibial lacerations

These injuries are particularly common in elderly women. The skin of the shin is thin, with a poor blood supply, due to the lack of underlying muscles. The worst situation of all is a distally-based flap at the junction of the middle and lower thirds of the shin, in a patient taking steroids. It is a general rule of medicine that, if there are a number of commonly employed treatments for the same condition, none of the treatments is particularly reliable: this applies to pretibial lacerations. Plastic surgeons tend to advocate radical surgery as an in-patient (Jones, B. M. and Sanders, R. (1983). Pretibial injuries: a common pitfall. *British Medical Journal*, **286**, 502), whereas accident and emergency consultants tend to a more conservative approach (Marsden, A. K. and Christian, M. S. (1983). Correspondence. *British Medical Journal*, **286**, 800–1). My own practice is as follows:

- Warn the patient that the injury will take 'weeks or months' to heal
- Clean the flap and remove any obviously non-viable tissue
- Lay the flap flat, using adhesive skin-closure strips to oppose the skin edges, avoiding all tension; do not be too concerned if the skin edges fail to meet; I rarely if ever suture these injuries, as the sutures almost invariably pull through, leaving an even larger area to heal
- Apply an Ichthopaste bandage (see **Bandages**)
- Inspect the wound every 7 days initially and every 2 weeks when it is becoming under control; obviously more often if the patient is concerned (e.g. by increasing pain, suggesting infection); too frequent changes of dressings disturb the healing process to no purpose
- Stress and stress again the necessity of elevation of the leg above the horizontal when sitting; encourage the patient to walk

Nail in board penetrating sole

Every case should be given intramuscular or oral antibiotics and tetanus toxoid antigen as indicated.

Fork through foot

Treat as above, for the same reasons. Exploration of severely contaminated wounds is needed.

Ruptured plantaris tendon (so-called)

A minor injury with surprisingly major symptoms. There is a characteristic history of sudden pain during active contraction; often bruising and tenderness develop just above the maximum girth of the calf. Treatment consists of support, and crutches if necessary. It is painful for about 10 days. The pathology of the condition is much disputed, but whether it is a torn vein (bruising may be severe), a muscular tear of gastrocnemius, or whatever, it is a recognizable syndrome with a label which makes the sufferer feel safer, and management more confident.

Traumatic arthrosis

Following sprains and blows, especially in the elderly, support and anti-inflammatory agents for a short period (5–10 days) are helpful.

Ruptured biceps (long head)

This is spontaneous, in elderly men as a rule, presenting with a painless lump in the upper arm. Symptomatic treatment with physiotherapy is usually sufficient.

Blanket gangrene

This is not uncommon in babies who wriggle their toes. Strands of wool, cotton, or synthetic fibres encircle the toes (fingers rarely), are pulled tight, produce oedema and circulatory occlusion; eventually gangrene. Treatment is only effective if a longitudinal linear incision down to bone is made in the affected digit. Relief is rapid. Choose a plane without crucial structures in it. Give antibiotics as common sense suggests.

Bites of tongue

These are very common in children. Do not suture unless there is uncontrollable bleeding or gross dehiscence. Sutures in the mouth are uncomfortable and inefficient, and generally become infected. If you have to stitch, use 4/0 or 5/0 Dexon. Give antibiotics and frequent mouth-washes. See also **Dental, miscellaneous**.

■ Intussusception

This should be considered in every vomiting child under the age of 5 in the presence of colic and the absence of diarrhoea. Red currant jelly on the tip of the examining finger is a positive confirmation but its absence is not significant. Admit for observation or urgent surgery.

■ Knee

The diagnosis of knee injuries is difficult. An accurate history of the injury and the immediate progress thereafter is mandatory. Initial examination is hampered by pain and swelling. Regardless of the particular injury sustained, it is essential that attention is paid to the quadriceps musculature from the patient's first visit, as wasting can occur very rapidly and good muscles are necessary to exert a protective effect to the injured joint; mobilization of the joint and/or static exercises are

required and physiotherapy is most important. Different orthopaedic surgeons have different ideas and you must always try to treat in the way they prefer; some like to deal with knee disorders from the beginning and may wish to perform examination under anaesthesia and/or arthroscopy.

Acute effusion

This may be due to traumatic synovitis or to haemorrhage. Simple effusions are cool and develop over 24 hours or so; haemorrhagic ones are hot, more painful, and develop more rapidly. Aspirate the really tense ones via the suprapatellar pouch, lateral approach, under full aseptic precautions; apply a pressure bandage after aspiration. Review the patient after 2 or 3 days, by which stage diagnosis will be a little easier. Haemarthrosis can occur without apparent structural damage to the knee, especially in the elderly and arthritic; but assume that there is structural damage until the contrary is proved. If blood is withdrawn leave it to stand; a supernatant layer of fat globules is very suggestive of bony injury even if X-ray is negative. Pyogenic arthritis needs emergency admission (cf. **Musculoskeletal emergencies**).

Internal derangement of the knee

Localize the injury by examination. If the knee is locked, give intramuscular pethidine 100 mg, and see if the rest will straighten the knee. If genuine locking occurs, which is fairly rare, manipulate under intravenous midazolam (see **Dislocations**) or general anaesthesia. In order to exclude the presence of a loose body you need anteroposterior and lateral radiographs with oblique, tunnel, and skyline views as well; these may also disclose, for example, osteochondritis dissecans of the medial femoral condyle. A plaster of Paris cylinder or pressure bandage gives support and confidence after reduction. If either of the collateral ligaments or either of the cruciates have been damaged, a pressure bandage will suffice until the morning, unless the knee is unstable when admission will

Lumps in the popliteal fossa

*
*
*

■ Hypothermia

be necessary. A plaster of Paris cylinder with weight-bearing for 10 days to 3 weeks is the definitive treatment for injury to either collateral ligament.

Repair is needed for collateral ligaments which are ruptured, as estimated by instability of the joint on stress; pain on stress is usually absent if rupture is complete. Partial meniscectomy is usually performed arthroscopically nowadays (Gallannaugh, S. C. (1986). Arthroscopic surgery of the knee. *British Medical Journal*, **293**, 710–11).

Lumps in the popliteal fossa

- **Semimembranosus bursa** Medial
- **Baker's cyst** Degenerative, with arthritis; usually midline
- **Popliteal aneurysm** Pulsatile

■ Laryngostomy

This is an invaluable emergency operation which is very rarely necessary except in cases of mandibular fracture associated with injury to the floor of the mouth. Still more rarely it may have to be resorted to in cases of asphyxia where intubation proves impossible. It is done as follows:

1. Palpate the cricothyroid ligament with one finger.
2. Make a *transverse* skin incision over it, 2.5 cm wide.
3. Clean the cricothyroid ligament by blunt dissection with a dry gauze swab.
4. Press the sharp end of a number 15 scalpel blade through the ligament so as to make a *vertical* slit.
5. Insert a medium-sized disposable tracheostomy tube (Portex 27 French gauge) through the slit and tie the tapes round the neck—or a child's inflatable endotracheal tube which, with any luck, will allow positive-pressure ventilation.
6. Secure haemostasis by pressure or rarely by the use of clamps—this is the last item; oxygen, suction, and anaesthesia can follow through the airway thus provided as the occasion demands.

Provided laryngostomy is not maintained for more than 48 hours, and provided the cricothyroid ligament is opened with a *vertical* incision, subsequent difficulty with phonation is said to be entirely avoided. Every casualty officer should be expert at this operation and able to perform it in under 2 minutes, if required.

■ Lumbago

This is a name given to the following clinical syndrome: characteristically the complainant is fairly young, the onset of lumbar pain is sudden and unrelated to injury, and there is spasm of the lumbar muscles, which typically begins with a trivial action, such as stooping to pick something up. Cases of lumbago often present themselves as 'back injuries' and are all too often accepted as such. The history is crucial.

The pathogenesis of such lesions is unknown and will probably remain so. It is sometimes said that they are due to interfacetal connective tissue disorders in the lumbar spine: this cannot be disproved.

The treatment is simple where muscle spasm is severe: an intramuscular non-steroidal anti-inflammatory agent, e.g. diclofenac (Voltarol) 75 mg. Once this has been done it is possible to assess straight-leg raising reliably, and so differentiate from a true prolapsed intervertebral disc, and to perform such manipulations as may seem desirable to overcome or alleviate the underlying condition. Subsequent treatment should consist of: non-steroidal anti-inflammatory agents and analgesics by mouth; reasonably brief rest, using floor or fracture boards if pain is severe; physiotherapy, especially dorso-lumbar extension exercises: these are essential, as good muscle tone is the best prophylactic against recurrence. If the condition is associated with well-marked local tenderness in, for example, an interspinous ligament or muscular insertion, generous infiltration of the tender area with local lignocaine 1% and/or bupivacaine (Marcain) 0.5% can give dramatic relief.

If the syndrome does not approximate to the above description, other possible sources of pain should be investigated and eliminated. The above treatment gives excellent and rapid relief if used appropriately. If it is not successful, further radiological, haematological, and physical examination is required.

If investigation leaves the patient with pain but without specific diagnosis, **manipulation** (q.v.) under anaesthesia is often effective.

■ Major disasters

These may descend upon a hospital with minimal notice. Aircraft and train accidents can bring overwhelming numbers of casualties, and so can football crowds and terrorist attacks by fire or explosives.

There is no way of making adequate preparation and the more complicated a provisional plan is the greater the confusion that will ensue.

The essential features of any plan are:

1 The recipient of the alert (the telephonist?) should have a short-list of key people to tell.
2 The key people need a short-list of the second echelon to tell. All these people need to know beforehand in writing what their duties are.
3 Ward space has to be cleared.

Apart from communications, the aim of forward planning should be to prevent chaos by appointing one person to receive and document casualties as they arrive (usually the A & E consultant or his deputy), an experienced surgeon to establish priorities for treatment, and a reliable physician to deal with medical emergencies. The next aim is to allot one junior doctor and one nurse to each major casualty for resuscitation and supervision and hope that there are enough surgeons available to do the necessary operating.

Anything beyond this is trimming.

■ Malaria

Plasmodium falciparum infection may present as an acute pyrexial emergency with collapse, delirium, coma, splenomegaly, and hepatomegaly. The history may be confused by prolongation of the incubation period (normally 3 weeks) owing to drug prophylaxis. Emergency treatment consists of prompt intravenous saline infusion and admission for continued supportive care and specific chemotherapy. Thick and thin blood films should be made on reception, to identify the parasite.

Treatment and prophylaxis change frequently and depend on the area of the world and local sensitivities. Consult the local specialist.

Useful telephone numbers:

The Liverpool School of Tropical Medicine
051-708-9393

The London (St. Pancras) Hospital for Tropical
  Diseases   01-387-4411

East Birmingham Hospital   021-772-4311

■ Manipulation

This consists of two kinds:

Diagnostic

This is well exemplified by the painful knee in which specific diagnosis may be impossible because of pain and muscle spasm. General anaesthesia gives relaxation so that *gentle* manipulation can identify crepitus, locking, clicking, instability, and abnormal movement. Then a reasonable attempt at diagnosis can be made.

Therapeutic

This is applicable to a variety of A & E presentations, especially necks, backs, and knees, not to mention a wide variety of **dislocations** (q.v.).

Once a careful history and relevant investigations have established the absence of significant musculoskeletal disorder, or mere stiffness, as a source of pain and disability, whether due to trauma, disuse, misuse, or some other obscure (possibly psychogenic) cause, *manipulation* by experienced hands can give rapid and effective relief. It is an art more than a science and better taught by apprenticeship than reading, but has to be controlled by reason and appropriate scepticism. Success depends on knowing what you are at, being clear about your aim, and understanding from experience how much force to use.

If you manipulate a severely spondylitic spine, acute supraspinatus syndrome, vertebral Pott's disease, unstable dislocation, or some other risky pathological state, you will richly deserve the heavy damages that will be given against you in court.

The essence of a therapeutic manipulation is the enforcement of maximal movement of the relevant joints so as to relieve their stiffness and increase their mobility. Relaxation of muscle spasm shortly ensues.

■ Mistakes, some common

Mistakes are made in A & E units, as elsewhere, and it is important that we recognize them, learn from them, and avoid them in the future. Weekly meetings can include five minutes for audit, so that we can learn from other people's mistakes, before making them ourselves. Remember that good judgement is based on experience; experience is based on bad judgement.

You will be very hard put to make a mistake which has never been made before, or even one which your consultant has never seen (or made himself) before.

Below are a few which seem to occur with depressing frequency: *look them up*: if you can survive six months as a casualty officer without making any of these, you are very good, or very lucky, or not seeing enough patients.

- Failure to recognize a posterior dislocation of the shoulder on X-ray
- Failure to recognize a dislocated lunate on X-ray
- Failure to recognize a depressed fracture of the tibial plateau on X-ray
- Failure to recognize a calcaneal fracture on X-ray
- Failure to recognize a greenstick fracture on X-ray
- Failure to recognize a skull fracture on X-ray
- Failure to recognize a facial fracture on X-ray
- Failure to recognize a pneumothorax on X-ray
- Failure to distinguish a bipartite patella from a fracture on X-ray
- Failure to X-ray for an intra-ocular foreign body after hammering
- Failure to recognize a scaphoid fracture clinically
- Failure to recognize a fractured radial head or neck clinically
- Failure to recognize tendon and nerve injuries in the hand clinically
- Failure to recognize the rotational element of a spiral fracture of a finger clinically
- Blind clamping of a bleeding radial or ulnar artery
- Ill-advised attempt to remove a foreign body from the soft tissues

X-rays showing examples of the above radiological problems should be available in the department for consultation at all times.

Cf. **Complaints**

■ Multiple injuries

See **Accidents, major**

■ Musculoskeletal emergencies

These are mostly dealt with under separate headings; for individual conditions see **Index**.

Painful shoulder

Shoulder pain is a rotten pain, and the end result of severe shoulder pain is all too often a 'frozen' one. Careful differential diagnosis and early treatment should go far to prevent this.

Arthritis, osteo-   Keep it moving by support, encouragement, physiotherapy, and anti-inflammatory drugs.

Arthritis, pyogenic   Needs drainage, antibiotics, and punctilious after-care. Even so, since it occurs usually in the elderly and debilitated, a stiff joint is often the outcome.

Rotator cuff syndrome may follow a fall, a minor strain, or even come out of the blue. It is an acute synovitis/capsulitis involving the tendons of the rotator cuff which surround the shoulder joint and constitute the greater part of its structure. Rest, anti-inflammatory drugs and mobilization from the third or fourth day may produce mobility; if not, early intra-articular steroid injection should be given.

Supraspinatus syndrome is a localized variety of the above and merits a similar approach. It is characterized by the 'painful arc' on abduction, or, if severe, by loss of abduction. If there is accompanying calcification of the tendon a course of non-steroidal anti-inflammatory drugs should follow the intra-articular injection of methyl-prednisolone (Depo-Medrone), 40 mg.

Frozen shoulder is an adhesive capsulitis characterized by severe pain on attempted external rotation of the humerus. Its course is benign but prolonged (3–12 months); intra-articular steroids are generally useless; oral non-steroidal anti-inflammatory drugs may help a bit. Maintaining morale is a problem in severe cases. It is not usually traumatic in origin.

Painful foot

Stress fracture (q.v.).

Morton's metatarsalgia An interdigital 'neuroma', activated by bilateral compression by the metatarsal heads. It may need surgery and is an orthopaedic problem.

Plantar fasciitis It is sometimes generalized but more often locally tender under the heel. Treat with foam padding in *both* shoes, anti-inflammatory drugs, or topical steroid injection, in sequence or together.

Hallux rigidus A degenerative consequence of a congenital abnormality of the first metatarsophalangeal joint. Exacerbation often follows trauma. Limitation of flexion more than extension. Flexion deformity occurs late. Recognition and palliative treatment allay anxiety, but orthopaedic surgery is often needed eventually.

Osteochondritis

Instances of this curious group of developmental disorders of bone often present primarily in the A & E department. They are probably determined by local varieties of vasculitis in growing bone and are mostly self-limiting. A few need treatment.

A list is a useful *aide-mémoire*, together with their eponyms as these are still generally in use.

- *Lunate*, Kienböck's: may lead to necrosis and the need for excision of the lunate
- *Hip*, Perthes' disease of: see **Hip syndrome, painful**
- *Knee*, osteochondritis of the femoral condyle: may present as a loose body after 'dissection' of the affected area of cartilage
- *Patella*, chondromalacia of: characteristically tender on grinding. Rest in a plaster of Paris cylinder. Surgery is rarely needed
- *Distal pole of patella*, Sinding Larsen–Johansson: symptomatic treatment only
- *Tibial tuberosity*, Osgood–Schlatter's: plaster of Paris cylinder, symptomatic treatment only

- *Navicular bone*, Köhler's: symptomatic treatment only
- *Heel*, Sever's: symptomatic treatment only by raising the heels
- *Metatarsal head*, Freiberg's: often needs excision
- *Vertebral bodies*, Scheuermann's

Osteochondritis dissecans can affect the elbow (capitulum), ankle (talus), or hip, but the medial femoral condyle is the most common site.

These conditions form a strange collection and may not all be causally related.

■ Myocardial infarction

1   Make a diagnosis. This is often difficult and not necessarily clinched by an ECG in the acute phase. A clinical hunch may be all you have: never ignore it. The classical symptoms include crushing central chest pain radiating into the neck and arms, breathlessness, anxiety, nausea, and vomiting. The patient is often cold, clammy, and cyanosed. Blood pressure may be high or low. Record the pulse and blood pressure, examine the heart and lungs, and note signs of heart failure. Attach the patient to a cardiac monitor, do an ECG, and take bloods for full blood count, urea and electrolytes, glucose, cholesterol, and enzymes (creatine kinase, aspartate aminotransferase, lactate dehydrogenase, and myoglobin). A chest X-ray will be required at a reasonably early stage.

2   Give oxygen and insert an in-dwelling intravenous cannula. Give diamorphine 5 mg intravenously (together with prochlorperazine 12.5 mg intramuscularly) for analgesia and sedation and its haemodynamic effects; repeat if necessary.

3   Send for a physician. The arrival of numerous ventricular extrasystoles is an indication for intravenous lignocaine at once: 100 mg bolus, followed by an infusion of 2 mg/kg/h. Reassurance, calmness, quiet, and sedation are mandatory. Atropine is effective for sinus bradycardia.

Ventricular arrhythmias are more safely dealt with by intravenous lignocaine, 100 mg in a bolus dose, than by the bewildering multitude of autonomic moderators which can, in inexpert hands, themselves cause arrhythmias and asystole; fashions in this field change so rapidly that it is wise to keep the current β-blockers and unblockers in the poisons cupboard for the use of visiting physicians. Pacing can be life-saving in extreme bradycardia of sudden onset. Trans-oesophageal pacing is quickest and safest in the A & E unit.

4 Transfer the patient to the coronary care unit as rapidly as is reasonably possible.

Pseudo-coronary Spontaneous rupture of the oesophagus while vomiting against a vigorously contracting crico-pharyngeal sphincter; perforation is usually 2 cm above the diaphragm into the pleural cavity; if higher, it can cause mediastinitis; an early sign is emphysema of the neck. Urgent radiological diagnosis and urgent surgery are required. First aid consists of urgent treatment for toxic shock with intravenous Haemaccel and intravenous antibiotics. Dopamine may be indicated.

Cf. **Cardiac arrest**

Nails, digital

Injuries

Crushing and laceration involving finger nails in particular can be misleading, as a simple cut or split in the nail may conceal important underlying injury to the nail bed or terminal phalanx. If there is any doubt the whole nail should be carefully dissected off the subjacent tissues and the damage properly inspected, assessed, and treated. Careful suture may be required, or even reconstruction, in order to avoid prolonged disability or later complications.

Ingrowing toe nail

This is a tiresome, common, and disabling complaint attributable partly to tight footwear (socks as well as shoes), partly to bad nail care, and partly to congenital conformations of the toe conducive to this disorder.

Recurrent affliction should be dealt with by preventative packing of the corners of the growing nail so as to lift it over the paronychial pads, careful trimming of the nail so that it ends in a strictly horizontal edge, and, if nothing else will serve, extirpation of the germinal layer by careful carbolization of the ungual matrix. This must be done using liquefied phenol B.P. for 3 minutes and close attention to detail is essential. The method is safe, effective, relatively painless, and quick to heal. It needs to be done directly after removing the nail and in a bloodless field. Wash off the phenol with plenty of 70% isopropyl alcohol solution. This procedure replaces the tiresome and inefficient methods of surgical extirpation of the matrix.

Unilateral ingrowth is dealt with by unilateral resection of one quarter of the nail and carbolization; bilateral ingrowth by bilateral resection of one quarter of the nail and carbolization. Total ablation remains as the only cure for cylindronychia, pachyonychia, and onychogryphosis.

Subungual haematoma

The treatment is paracentesis unguis, with a paper-clip and spirit lamp. Subsequent dressings are required to mop up slow leakage of haematoma, which often persists for 48 hours. Relief is usually immediate. If it remains painful after paracentesis, look for a fracture of the terminal phalanx.

Subungual foreign body

See **Foreign bodies**

■ Necks

Acute neck pain, often with signs of root irritation, is a common emergency. Cf. **Torticollis, acute**.

Whiplash injury

This usually follows a road traffic accident. The characteristic symptoms (which may be delayed for 24 hours) are pain in the neck, which may radiate to the shoulder and arm or to the occiput, and stiffness. The neck is tender with a reduced range of movement. X-ray often shows an abnormally straight neck, due to muscle spasm. Treatment consists of a hard collar, analgesia, and physiotherapy as early as possible. Symptoms can continue for up to three years but usually eventually disappear completely.

Occipital neuralgia

This is a common consequence of whiplash injuries and blows to the head. The chief symptom is persistent headache, unrelieved by analgesics. Tenderness on local pressure over the greater occipital nerve is diagnostic. Manipulation under general anaesthesia, after X-ray, gives early relief; forced rotation is the key manipulation. Ultrasound or heat may be helpful.

Cervical spondylosis

This can accompany any of the acutely painful necks and sets a problem to the manipulator. If it is severe enough to threaten the stability of the spine, firm support is the only treatment. Experience and orthopaedic consultation must decide.

Cervical prolapsed intervertebral disc

See **Neuropathies**

■ Negligence

See **Complaints** and **Mistakes, some common**

■ Neurological emergencies

Rarely a therapeutic commitment to A & E units, but it's as well to identify the varieties and treat the treatable with understanding.

Cerebrovascular accidents

These may require airway care or intubation. Oxygen should always be given, as for head injuries.

Cerebral haemorrhage/thrombosis/embolism

Subarachnoid haemorrhage There is sudden severe headache, vomiting, photophobia, irritability, and clouding of consciousness, associated with neck rigidity and blood in the cerebrospinal fluid. Find out the local policy about intravenous tranexamic acid (Cyklokapron) as prophylaxis in this disaster.

Extradural or subdural haemorrhage

Acute extradural haematoma, from leakage from the middle meningeal vessels, is identified by local swelling, radiological fracture, dilatation of the ipsilateral pupil, increasing headache, and irritability giving way to coma. A lucid interval is common. The patient is usually below the age of 45 years and the prognosis is fairly good. *This is an absolute emergency.*

Chronic subdural haematoma, from lacerations of the venous sinuses, is typically associated with a fluctuating level of consciousness, but the overall trend is downwards. There are progressive signs of rising intracranial pressure. The patient is usually elderly or an alcoholic.

Generally there is considerable brain damage and the prognosis is relatively poor. This is a relative emergency.

Expert neurosurgical advice is needed.

Cf. **Head injuries**

Pyogenic conditions

Cerebral thrombophlebitis E.g. cavernous sinus thrombosis, spreading from a pararhinal boil or angular stomatitis. It is associated with general septicaemia or pyogenic conditions.

Brain abscess This may mimic an acute confusional state or a neoplasm.

Primary infections

- *Pyogenic meningitis*
- *Viral meningitis*
- Early *poliomyelitis* in the invasive stage
- *Encephalitis*: bizarre visual phantasies
- *Tabetic crises*: severe fleeting pains in the limbs or abdomen; Argyll–Robertson pupils and syphilitic neuropathy

Neoplasm

Haemorrhagic or oedematous crises can occur. A preceding history of cerebral disturbance may be absent.

Miscellaneous

- *Herxheimer reaction* from treatment of active syphilis
- *Myasthenic crisis*
- *Guillain–Barré syndrome*: an immunologically determined polyneuritis going on to
- *Bulbar palsy*

- *Acute vertigo*: viral (labyrinthitis)/acoustic neuroma/idiopathic: if you treat this with prochlorperazine (Stemetil), do not forget that this can produce acute extrapyramidal symptoms, usually facial athetosis, which can be reversed by benztropine (Cogentin) and withdrawal of the prochlorperazine.

Myopathy is not primarily an A & E concern but can present with an acute respiratory crisis due to choking, respiratory insufficiency, or injury. Treatment is by common sense application of routine measures.

■ Neuropathies

Various kinds may present in A & E units from long tract lesions (multiple sclerosis and syringomyelia) to motor neurone disease and amyotrophic lateral sclerosis, but their emergencies are incidental rather than accidental.

Prolapsed intervertebral disc

The commonest neuropathies seen are those arising from spondylotic changes and intervertebral disc lesions. Cervical and lumbar disc calamities often present as 'injuries' but a careful history discloses a practically spontaneous onset in a majority.

Acute cervical disc lesions with root signs (pain) but no muscle weakness are often effectively relieved by the following regime:

- Hard collar by day, properly applied
- Soft collar by night, properly applied
- Analgesics for one week
- Rest for one week
  followed if needed by:
- Cervical traction and/or manipulation
- Continued support

Gradual weaning from the use of collars is important.

Lumbar disc lesions can be identified by limitation of straight leg raising and their progress monitored by observing its recovery. Rest in bed for three weeks on fracture boards is good treatment but limiting. Plaster of Paris jackets may take 10 days to give relief but are very good in the long run and permit busy people to keep working. Temporary lumbo-sacral supports (e.g. Remploy) can be very useful in less severe or recurrent cases.

Cf. **Backs**

Rarely central disc prolapse can cause acute retention of urine.

Not every case needs full orthopaedic investigation and support, and those that do may well find it difficult to obtain. Orthopaedic consultation may however be necessary and must not be forgotten.

Careful examination, X-ray, and regard to the therapeutic outcome offer early relief to people suffering from a wretchedly painful and disabling complaint. These cases are well within the capacity of any painstaking General Practitioner but unfortunately the therapeutic facilities seldom are—one reason why the national average for annual increase of attendances at accident units in Britain stands at 10 per cent!

Cf. **Lumbago**

Saturday night palsy

Radial palsy due to compression of the radial nerve in its sulcus on the humerus, historically attributed to falling into a drunken stupor with the gloriously relaxed arm flopping over the arm of a chair. It can also occur at the axillary level in the same way (cf. 'crutch palsy'). It is treated by the use of a 'lively' splint and may take weeks or months to recover.

Bell's palsy

The onset is painless and sudden.

Cf. **Viruses**

Zoster of the geniculate ganglion (Ramsay–Hunt syndrome)

Look for the tympanic vesicles which soon merge into a general tympanitis. There is generally pain before palsy. Treat with adrenocorticotrophic hormone 40 international units daily or at 48-hour intervals. Acyclovir may help.

Cf. **Viruses**

Acute eighth nerve palsy (viral)

See **Ear, nose, and throat emergencies**

Thoracic outlet syndrome

Nerve root compression by cervical rib, fibrous band, or clavicle on first rib (shopping bag palsy); it is also common in pregnancy. A sling gives first aid relief. It is characterized by aching pain (worse by day) in the early stages, and interosseous wasting later.

Other tunnel syndromes

Elbow Anterior and posterior interosseous nerves; ulnar nerve.

Carpal tunnel syndrome Median nerve pain in the palm, spreading up the forearm; worse at night. Relieved by night splintage. May need surgery.

Popliteal tunnel syndrome Intermittent claudication in young soldiers.

Anterior and posterior tibial compartment syndromes Rare and needing surgery.

Meralgia paraesthetica Lateral cutaneous nerve of thigh compressed at the pelvic brim or in the muscle belly of sartorius. May need a surgical remedy.

Peroneal palsy Surgical remedy.

■ News media

Always respect the patient's confidentiality; the media know you have no other choice. But remember that the gentlemen of the press have a job to do and that they can be very useful allies. The local newspaper and radio almost always prefer to support hospital staff—the doctors and nurses anyway—than to criticize them, and the same is often true of the national press and television. Cultivate them today and they may be able and willing to help you tomorrow.

Make provision for them in the event of a major incident; they will be there whether you like it or not, and will be contented with a steady supply of drink and information.

■ Nomenclature

In an accident department, cases are continually passed from one doctor to another and accurate labelling is important and time-saving. This is particularly true when medical reports have to be made in the absence of the patient and after the relevant doctor has left. Incidentally, if your labelling is accurate your diagnosis is likely to be the same. When in doubt refer to *Gray's anatomy* (see **Bibliography**).

Fingers

As there is no consistency in the numbering of the digits it is easiest to use their names:

Thumb
Index
Middle
Ring
Little

It has been known for judges in court to become very savage with opposing medical witnesses who refer to the 'second' and 'third' fingers, when they both intend to refer to the identical digit.

■ Nursing services

The success of the A & E enterprise is dependent on the skill and quality as much of its nursing staff as of its medical staff. The relationship between them is important. In most departments (unless they are attached to a teaching hospital which supplies students in quantity) experienced nurses need to take a large share of daily routine work. As well as dressings and general organization they often undertake suturing, venepuncture, cardiography, catheterization, monitoring, plastering, and even intubation. Very well they do them too. It has to be remembered that procedures outside their general training remain the responsibility of the medically qualified staff, but nevertheless they are done to a standard which equals that of the medical staff. Nurses' training in these extra tasks is the responsibility of the senior medical staff and no pains are too great to be expended on it. The doctors will, of course, gain greatly from the nurses' skills, but the chief beneficiaries will be the injured. Distinction of function between nursing and medical staffs (but *not* distinction of responsibility) rapidly becomes blurred in accident work, and the more blurred, the better the department works. It is important for all parties in the team to work actively towards a relationship of constructive harmony.

Experienced casualty nurses, of all grades, are a breed apart: tough yet sympathetic, resilient yet able to accept constructive criticism, enthusiastic and energetic, yet able to relax when the opportunity arises. Their knowledge is profound and they are willing to teach you, but they are also keen to learn and try new techniques. Their sense of responsibility is matched only by their sense of humour. They are worth their weight in gold.

■ Obstetric emergencies

In countries where hospitals are far apart and medical services thinly spread, any obstetric emergency can arrive. Ideally an obstetrician should always be available to deal with impacted labours, maternal or fetal distress, major obstetric haemorrhages, malpresentations, and fetal deformities. In fact accident surgeons will have been conditioned by experience to cope when they are unsupported.

Any experienced accident surgeon or casualty officer should be prepared to do an instant Caesarean section to extract a live baby from a mother in the last trimester of pregnancy, killed in a road traffic accident. Thereafter the problem is one of ordinary infant resuscitation, warming, and disposal to an appropriate baby unit. The practical problems and pitiful heartbreak which ensue are not the casualty officer's problem.

Accidental haemorrhage (concealed or revealed) and haemorrhage due to placenta praevia may also arrive at our door and may need intravenous analgesia and the institution of resuscitation by intravenous infusion before being sent to a specialist unit. The casualty officer's response will be determined by the time-lag involved in the transfer. If there is far to go or a long delay in getting there, blood transfusion should be started and the obstetric flying squad called or urgent transfer arranged, accompanied by a doctor.

Precipitate delivery and post-partum haemorrhage may arrive urgently at an A & E department. Syntometrine (ergometrine maleate 500 μg + oxytocin 5 U) is the best emergency drug and should be given intramuscularly after the delivery of the anterior shoulder. It should also be given intravenously for post-partum bleeding without attempting to identify or remove retained placenta.

Eclampsia This is a fulminating hypertension of pregnancy with proteinuria and presenting with fits. Treatment consists of an intravenous anticonvulsant, such as diazepam, and urgent specialist management. If transfer to another hospital is necessary, the patient

Obstructed labour

should be accompanied by a doctor, after the blood pressure has been lowered with intravenous hydralazine.

Incarcerated retrogravid uterus is usually associated with acute retention of urine. Catheterize; possibly replace in anteversion if specialized help is distant.

Prolapsed cord Put the patient into the Trendelenburg position to elevate the pelvis. Urgent referral to a specialist unit is required.

Cf. **Abortions**

■ Oesophageal occlusion

This is a common A & E calamity, because it is of sudden onset (though possibly preceded by dysphagia), often brings great discomfort, and is always frightening. Retrosternal pain may be low (achalasia or neoplasm), middle (mediastinal new growth), or high (oesophageal pouches and diverticula).

The neoplastic and neuromuscular causes of this condition are obvious, but the 'greedy old man' syndrome is less well known, although much commoner. It consists in swallowing unchewed lumps of meat (usually) which the elderly oesophagus cannot transmit. Generally they soften physiologically and pass on their way. Sometimes they have to be extricated by way of an oesophagoscope. Some swear by the efficacy of passing a nasogastric tube or a small balloon catheter which can pass the obstruction and then be withdrawn after inflating the balloon; this then acts as an extractor. Such remedies may well be of use in the absence of a capable gastroscopist but could well do irrevocable damage to an oesophagus obstructed by stricture or neoplasm. The prevention of recurrence is not by admonition but by mincing all meat.

Pouches and diverticula can occlude the gullet by simply filling slowly with food, drink, and spittle until nothing more can get by. Regurgitation may relieve the blockage, but oesophagoscopy and repair may be required.

■ Pain

This used to be the physician's first enemy, but death has displaced it. In general pethidine is excellent: 100 mg intramuscularly for an adult. If the patient is shocked, give pethidine in small frequent doses intravenously, the dose and frequency titrated by the effect: if it were given intramuscularly, it could have minimal effect (and perhaps be repeated) until tissue perfusion improved, when a bolus could suddenly enter the circulation. The injection will often make proper examination of the injured and frightened patient possible, when without it it was impossible. Naloxone 0.8 mg, repeated if necessary, reverses respiratory depression. Some surgeons are annoyed when patients are given this necessary relief, but the damage is to their *amour propre*, and not to the certain diagnosis of the patient's disease or injury.

Entonox (a 50:50 mixture of O_2 and N_2O) should be available in every A & E department and can be used freely without risk. Many ambulances carry it and it can be used effectively for patients in pain during their journey. It is good for painful dressings after surgery or injury.

Use a few analgesics of varying strengths, from paracetamol to diamorphine, and get to know them well.

■ Physiotherapy

This is a hospital department which has its own expertise and pride and should never be used as a dump for patients in whom you have failed to make a diagnosis or cure.

Physiotherapists have special skills (e.g. manipulations), special tools (e.g. ultrasound), and inexhaustible patience. They can and do help greatly with sprained ankles, acute spinal disorders including whiplash injuries, hand injuries, rehabilitation of patients whose injuries have been treated by immobilization, and a multitude of other problems. They also have an invaluable contribution to make in helping the frightened and hurt to use

joints which have become stiff and painful for a variety of reasons, and only need movement to make them comfortable and effective once again. In general, the earlier they see a patient, the better for all concerned. They are an integral part of the accident family and appreciate being consulted, shown films of injuries, and being asked for advice. Their role can be improved and enhanced by their being included in relevant **clinical trials** (q.v.).

■ 'Plasma expanders'

In cases of blood loss you often need to use a 'plasma expander' to fill the gap until blood becomes available. While you are wondering which to use put up 500 ml of normal saline, which cannot do any harm unless the patient is in congestive cardiac failure. Electrolyte solutions (normal saline and Ringer's lactate) only stay in the intravascular compartment for a short time and so cannot be used to replace lost blood volume. A 'plasma expander' is required for this.

There are three choices: human Plasma Protein Fraction (supplied by the Blood Transfusion Service), which is costly and not really appropriate for simple blood loss; an inert polysaccharide (Dextran 70); or a gelatin solution (Haemaccel and Gelofusine).

Human Plasma Protein Fraction should be kept for patients with plasma loss (i.e. extensively burnt patients), and the dextrans have the disadvantage of interfering with blood cross-matching, preventing normal clotting and bleeding mechanisms from working effectively, and, by producing extracellular fluid retention, causing pulmonary oedema.

The gelatin solutions have none of these snags, have a short half-life (4 hours), are diuretic, and produce no ill effects on normal clotting and bleeding mechanisms. They are made from degraded beef gelatin (which produces a short-chain molecule) and are not antigenic. The anaphylactoid reactions to these solutions occasionally reported in the medical press are said to be due to

increased histamine production; they can be treated by stopping the infusion and giving antihistamines.

In use Haemaccel has proved effective and trouble-free and is therefore the 'plasma expander' of choice. Incidentally, it is not very expensive, has a shelf-life of 8 years, and is unaffected by freezing or tropical temperatures.

Do not forget that blood loss of more than about 2 litres needs urgent replacement by blood. Nothing else will do.

Cf. **Shock, surgical**

■ Plaster of Paris

The application of plaster of Paris is learnt by apprenticeship, not by reading. Other materials can be used: some are lighter, some stronger, some more radiolucent, some dry more rapidly, some do not disintegrate in water.

Swelling of a limb is inevitable after injury and the great danger of a plaster lies in the fact that it forms a rigid casing, so that if swelling occurs within it the circulation of the limb is endangered. Precautions must be taken to prevent this; if it should occur the signs must be recognized and corrective action taken immediately: removing or splitting the plaster.

Whereas a full plaster of Paris completely encircles the limb, a slab covers only part of the circumference of the limb so that swelling of the limb is less likely to endanger the circulation. A slab can be removed more easily and more rapidly than a full plaster in an emergency. An alternative method of reducing the danger of swelling is to split the plaster down to the skin along its length after application.

A slab is thus preferable to a full plaster during the first two or three days after injury, when swelling is likely to be increasing.

A patient who is allowed home after application of a plaster should be provided with verbal and written instructions regarding his plaster, and particularly regarding the possibility of swelling, and by giving the

instruction. Suitable plaster instructions given below.

Plaster Instructions

1. Return to hospital immediately if limb bluish or becomes cold, swollen, very painful, very white, stiff, red, or begins to itch.

2. Elevate the injured or casted surface (e.g. on pillow or sling) as much as possible for the first 2 days at least.

3. Plaster of Paris takes at least 36 hours to dry — do not bear weight on the plaster during this time.

4. Keep the plaster dry.

5. Return to hospital if the plaster changes or becomes loose.

6. Remove the limit of the cast and do all work included in the plaster.

Pneumothorax

Pneumonia

See Chest injuries

Spontaneous

In the young. This is common in otherwise well young adults linked to ... The chest showing ... towards the base. There may be considerable ... respiratory distress as the vital return of muscle that ... rapidly. Both inspiration and expiration ... this ... should be taken. Percutaneous aspiration or subsequent ... pneumothorax recurs below a ... out on the ... intervention is then required.

In the elderly, rupture of emphysematous bullae is a cause of pneumothorax. These are rather easier to diag-

regarding the possibility of swelling endangering the circulation. Suitable plaster instructions are given below.

Plaster instructions

1. Return to hospital immediately if the hand/foot becomes blue, swollen, very painful, very cold, stiff, red, or begins to tingle.
2. Elevate the arm/leg on a soft surface (e.g. a pillow or sling) as much as possible for the first 3 days at least.
3. Plaster of Paris takes about 48 hours to dry: do not bear weight on the plaster during this time.
4. Keep the plaster dry.
5. Return to hospital if the plaster cracks or becomes loose.
6. Exercise the joints of the limb which are not included in the plaster.

◼ Pneumothorax

Traumatic

See **Chest injuries**

Spontaneous

In the young This is common after exertion and is characterized by sudden pain in the chest radiating towards the back. There may be considerable cardio-respiratory distress at the onset owing to mediastinal mobility. Both inspiratory and expiratory chest X-rays should be taken. Refer to the physicians for admission. Spontaneous resolution can occur but thoracic intubation is often required.

In the elderly Ruptured emphysematous bullae in cases of cor pulmonale may tip the balance of cardiac

sufficiency quite drastically and produce an acute cardio-respiratory emergency. Oxygen and paracentesis thoracis are needed for first aid, followed by admission, to the intensive care unit if respiratory embarrassment is severe.

Cf. **Thoracic intubation**

■ Poisoning

This is common in children by accident and in adults on purpose (see also **Psychiatric emergencies**). Management is basically simple as far as primary treatment goes; it consists essentially of:

1 Re-establishment of vital functions (intubation, intravenous infusion, cardiac support).
2 Removal of any poison that may still be in the stomach (stomach wash out or emesis): saline emetics must never be used as they are themselves electrolytically toxic and an occasional fatal result is reported, especially in children; syrup of ipecacuanha is the best emetic for general use.
3 Administration of a specific antidote if available.
4 Elimination of what has been absorbed.
5 Adsorption of poisons in the bowel where possible.
6 General supportive care.

Exceptions to these general rules are:

Corrosives, which must not be treated by gastric lavage or emesis, as they may well intensify the damage done to the oesophagus on the way down as they come up again, producing perforation where only ulceration had already occurred. Buffer solutions should be given either by mouth or by Ryle's tube: milk is the best, but ice cream is more acceptable to small children. If there is evidence of perforation already (great retrosternal pain and collapse) nothing must be given by mouth but refer the patient for immediate oesophagoscopy, etc.

Volatile hydrocarbons such as petrol, benzene, carbon tetrachloride, chloroform, and trichlorethylene should not be treated with whole milk as their absorption is

Obscure poisons

increased by the presence of fat in the small bowel. This probably applies to kerosene (commercial paraffin) as well. These should be treated with copious watery fluids or skim milk by mouth and *admission*, as toxic effects may be of late onset. The danger of inhalation of these agents during vomiting is of prime importance, so that stomach wash out and emesis are contra-indicated.

Children, in whom some consider that gastric lavage should never be used because of the stress and anxiety it causes them. Emesis should be obtained by giving ipeca-cuanha. Others do not entirely accept this view, at least in the case of iron or aspirin overdose. Iron, they hold, is so toxic that no delay in emptying the stomach is per-missible, and aspirin is notorious for causing pyloric spasm, which can delay absorption by as much as 12–24 hours, with possibly fatal delayed intoxication. This is a trap for the unwary.

Obscure poisons

These often set a problem of a particular kind because the agent may be unfamiliar both to you and to the toxico-logist; even direct reference to a manufacturer may produce no information whatever, or even that the product is of unknown constitution. A few suggestions on how to proceed may be useful in the circumstances, and the following approach is suggested:

1 At first contact (usually by telephone) insist that the container, contents, and any available maker's instructions are brought with the patient: this is very important and can easily save hours of further messing about.
2 Known pharmaceutical preparations and galenicals: refer to standard works such as the *British national formulary* or Matthew and Lawson, *Treatment of common acute poisonings* (see **Bibliography**).
3 Known agricultural poisons and sprays: identify in *Approved products for farmers and growers* (see **Bibliography**).

4   If no definite information is available look up in Gosselin, *Clinical toxicology of commercial products* (see **Bibliography**), identify the constituents of the poison, and refer to them in the appropriate sections.

5   Ordinary domestic preparations thought to be toxic: treat as 4.

6   Berries, flowers, and plants can be identified in Frohne and Pfänder's *A colour atlas of poisonous plants* (see **Bibliography**).

7   If all else fails ring one of the poisons centres (see below) and if necessary consult the toxicologist. These centres have a definite but limited usefulness: they can give helpful information in many cases, but cannot in general discuss problems of diagnosis and management. Their standards are high and information extensive. The responsibility for diagnosis and treatment remains, however, with the clinician.

8   Every accident department should keep a toxicology file to give access to up-to-date information.

Specific antidotes

Opiates: naloxone 0.4 mg intravenously repeated every 2 minutes or so until the desired effect is produced. It is also effective against dextropropoxyphene (Distalgesic), which causes respiratory depression.

Iron: desferrioxamine:

1   Take blood for serum iron.

2   Stomach wash out with desferrioxamine solution, 2 g/l of warm water, followed by the instillation of desferrioxamine 5 g into the stomach.

3   Give desferrioxamine 2 g intramuscularly at once (0.5 g for children under 2 years old, 1 g for children over 2 years old); intravenous desferrioxamine 5 mg/kg/h to a maximum of 80 mg/kg/day is also recommended; this is probably best dealt with after admission, together with monitoring of serum-free iron.

Heavy metals (lead, mercury, gold, arsenic, copper): dimercaprol should be available as an effective antidote, even though these poisons are rarely met and are unlikely to present as emergencies.

Paracetamol poisoning should be treated with gastric lavage if seen within 4 hours. When seen later than this, the plasma concentration of paracetamol should be measured; if the concentration falls above a line drawn between 1.32 mmol/l at 4 hours and 0.33 mmol/l at 15 hours after the overdose, acetylcysteine should be given intravenously; alternatively, methionine can be given orally unless the patient is vomiting or unconscious. Both these agents are of little value after 15 hours.

Patients at risk of hepatic failure should have a prophylactic infusion of dextrose to prevent hypoglycaemia, and established hepatic or renal failure is managed conventionally (Meredith, T. J., Prescott, L. F., and Vale, J. A. (1986). Why do patients still die from paracetamol poisoning? *British Medical Journal*, **293**, 345–6).

Phenothiazines (e.g. prochlorperazine): benztropine 1 mg intravenously, repeated as necessary, for extrapyramidal effects.

Tricyclic antidepressants can produce cardiac arrhythmias and cardiac monitoring is required.

Cyanide: Give intravenous chelating agent Co-EDTA (dicobalt edetate: Kelocyanor) 600 mg, followed by a further 300 mg 1 minute later if not effective; this is toxic and may induce collapse and vomiting for a brief period. Follow with 50 ml of 50% glucose intravenously. Alternatively, or if dicobalt edetate is ineffective, give 10 ml of sodium nitrite 3% slowly intravenously, followed by 25 ml of sodium thiosulphate 50% very slowly intravenously. These quasi-specific antidotes should be prominently displayed in the reception area as speed of treatment is of paramount importance.

General antidotes

Charcoal (activated and finely divided) can be given in water down a stomach tube as an adsorbent and is reputedly effective in reducing the absorption of **tricyclic antidepressants, paracetamol**, and other poisons.

Whole blood filtration through a charcoal column is recommended for **paraquat** and **diquat** poisoning, and is available at Guy's Hospital (01-407-7600), East Birmingham Hospital (021-772-4311), and other centres which may be nearer to you. It must be done as soon as the poison is identified in the urine, and if the patient is far away helicopter delivery is likely to be required if irreversible lung damage is to be avoided. If you have seen the utterly hideous consequences of paraquat poisoning you will readily agree to grasp at any straw which might deliver your patient from the delayed, horrific, and inevitable consequences of his folly or despair. Intravenous fluids should be started early to maintain the urinary output and so increase the excretion of paraquat (Williams, P. S., Hendy, M. S., and Ackrill, P. (1984). Early management of paraquat poisoning. *Lancet*, **i**, 627). **Fuller's earth** and **bentonite** are other adsorbent media which have been recommended for paraquat: 150 g in milk, water, or squash can be given at first contact without fear of harm and with possible benefit. Mannitol 20% is the vehicle currently recommended for fuller's earth; 200 ml given by naso-gastric tube; it is followed by magnesium sulphate by mouth to increase the excretion of adsorbed paraquat. Obtain a copy of *The treatment of paraquat poisoning*, available from ICI Central Toxicology Laboratories, Alderley Park, Macclesfield, Cheshire, SK10 4TJ (0625-582711).

Poisons centres

London	01-407-7600
Cardiff	0222-569200
Edinburgh	031-229-2477, ext. 2233
Belfast	0232-240503
Dublin	0001-745588

■ Press, the

See News media

■ Psychiatric emergencies

Acute confusion

Whether emotional, toxic, or senile in origin, should be left untreated if possible until seen by a psychiatrist. If not it is best controlled by intramuscular diazepam 10 mg, repeated if necessary; or, if the restlessness is combined with violence or dangerous wandering, paraldehyde 10 ml (not more than 5 ml at any one site) from a glass syringe may be needed. Drug addiction is a major factor in big cities.

Acute disturbance

Is generally of emotional origin associated with crises of bereavement, matrimony, or other close personal relationships; it can take many forms, such as withdrawal, disorientation, hysterical fugue with loss of memory, etc. These must be handled gently with understanding from the start. They do not need, as a rule, any emergency treatment, but gauche or insensitive handling in the A & E unit can increase the difficulties of all concerned to a serious degree. Drugs should be avoided in the A & E unit.

Acute mania

Is usually associated with organic mental illness: manic-depressive psychosis, schizophrenia, cerebral tumour, etc. Acute mania can be due to acute toxaemia (usually bacterial and post-operative) and to thyrotoxicosis (q.v.); recognition early is crucial as the cause needs treating more urgently than the symptoms. It is also common in alcoholism (acute withdrawal mania, i.e. delirium tremens) and drug addiction, either as part of a withdrawal

syndrome or as a toxic manifestation of drugs like lysergic acid diethylamide (LSD). Paraldehyde may be necessary to bring the situation under control, but more importantly large doses of chlorpromazine (50 mg intramuscularly, repeated if required) are needed. The earlier intravenous high-potency B vitamins are given in delirium tremens the better. An intravenous infusion of chlormethiazole (Heminevrin) 0.8%, 40–100 ml over 10 minutes then adjusted according to the response, is the current remedy for delirium tremens.

Psychopathy

Is a term applied to varieties of personality disorder which are a personal or social nuisance. Aggressive and manipulative psychopaths are the bane of accident units and are not usually violent. They require endless patience and skill to handle and are inaccessible to reasoning or pharmacy. The final resort is to ask for help from the police, who often know all about them. They can disrupt an entire department for long periods but seldom transgress the law.

Sociopathy

Is an etymologically bastard form of the above in which the personality defect expresses itself in an inability to fit in with social norms or to make ordinary provision for basic needs such as food, shelter, clothing, and care of children. Such people haunt hospitals demanding fares to non-existent relatives in remote towns and hope to be able to spend the proceeds on (for instance) booze. Social workers should cope with them but in fact, more often than not, lack the facilities to do so.

Attempted suicide

The medical problems (e.g. poisoning) or the surgical problems (e.g. cut throat or wrist) take immediate priority over the psychiatric aspects and the patient may well require admission under the care of the physicians or

surgeons. If not, a psychiatrist should be consulted before the patient is allowed home. Remember that the patient's pharmacological knowledge may be very limited and an overdose which is clearly not dangerous *per se* may nevertheless represent a very real attempt, which could be successfully repeated in another form. I personally do not subscribe to the belief that psychological as well as physical assessment may be carried out by junior doctors in A & E departments (Kessel, N. (1985). Patients who take overdoses. *British Medical Journal*, **290**, 1297–8), if only because they lack the time to do this properly.

Certification of the insane

The casualty officer lacks both the time and the expertise to deal with this situation: send for a psychiatrist. Avoid sedation if you can, so that the psychiatrist can draw his own conclusions from an unfuddled patient.

See also **Confusion, acute; Drug addiction** and **Drunkenness**

■ Pyrexia of unknown origin

Unravelling a pyrexia of unknown origin (PUO) is no part of the duties of a casualty officer but nonetheless patients do present with some frequency. They should not be sent away undiagnosed. History and examination may make some diagnoses more obvious (e.g. tuberculosis, mumps, Henoch–Schönlein purpura) while in others special investigations are required (e.g. glandular fever, malaria, carcinoma of the bronchus). If you can't make a diagnosis, refer to the physicians or paediatricians for their opinions. Remember that the elucidation of PUO has become much more difficult in these days of frequent inter-continental air travel.

■ Quinsy (peritonsillar abscess)

This is a very painful and distressing emergency treated as follows:

1 Give benzylpenicillin 600 mg or cephradine 500 mg intramuscularly at once.
2 Give surface anaesthesia to the pharynx with 10% lignocaine spray, the patient sitting up on the bed or trolley.
3 Make one stab in the area where the pus points, using a scalpel with a number 15 blade on it: let the patient cough and spit.
4 Open the incision widely with a small artery forceps.

Pus will pour out and the patient will be grateful for ever. Continue appropriate local bathing and systemic antibiotics. A good headlight is essential.

It may be that your consultant ENT surgeon will prefer to provide this treatment himself, but maybe not.

■ Rabies

Rabies is a neurotropic virus infection which is susceptible to treatment in the first few days but not afterwards. It can be transmitted by biting, licking, or the mere contamination of skin wounds or mucous membranes with infected saliva. The incubation period varies from 10 days to 20 years but is usually less than 1 month; the more peripheral the wound, the longer the incubation period. The terror which overwhelms people who think they have been exposed to infection is fully justified by the dreadful nature of the 'furious' form of the disease; the French *la rage* is a telling name.

It is important that every patient who presents with the possibility of a bite from a rabid animal should be treated seriously, and proper measures for protection and control taken. Infected domestic animals, especially dogs, are the main danger, but the infection can come from any warm-blooded animal outside the United Kingdom and Eire. The possibility that the patient has contracted rabies is

raised if the animal which bit him has died or disappeared or if the wound is dirty and contused. Foxes and vampire bats are the chief wild vectors.

The earliest symptoms are paraesthesiae at the site of the bite and failure of wound healing. Once hydrophobia and muscle spasm have set in the prognosis is virtually hopeless, but cases have been known to recover in intensive care as the virus ultimately loses its virulence.

Advice is immediately available from the Communicable Disease Surveillance Centre, Colindale, London (01-200-6868): they operate a 24-hour-per-day service and will be able to put you in touch with the nearest branch of the Public Health Laboratory Service (PHLS), who in turn will supply rabies vaccine. The vaccine should be given at the earliest possible opportunity. Human rabies immunoglobulin must be given in addition to vaccine in all cases where the risk of exposure is high. Early surgical excision of the wound, thorough irrigation, and sterilization with tincture of iodine are also needed. Routine tetanus prophylaxis may be required.

The Liverpool School of Tropical Medicine (051-708-9393) also provides a 24-hour-per-day service for advice.

■ Radiographers

Most radiographers are superb and thoroughly co-operative. If they are given requests which are specific and warranted by the clinical condition of the patient they can be magnificent. Often there is a radiographer on call who objects to being sent for: remind them that the clinical responsibility lies with the casualty officer, not the radiographer. Try to cultivate the radiographers, as they can be helpful in advising on views and diagnosing fractures on X-ray: but they are often reluctant to comment, which is a pity because their opinion is well worth having, although again the final responsibility is the doctor's — no one would deny this.

Cf. **X-rays**

■ Renal emergencies

See **Urogenital emergencies** and **Urogenital injuries**

■ Respiratory emergencies

Bronchial asthma

See **Asthma, bronchial**

Spontaneous pneumothorax

See **Pneumothorax**

Pneumonia or **bronchitis** in patients with pulmonary insufficiency (e.g. obstructive airways disease, pulmonary fibrosis, emphysema): give 24% oxygen by mask; measure the blood gases urgently and adjust the oxygen therapy according to the result; admit.

Bronchiolitis in infants: oxygen tent and steam.

Major haemoptysis: suction, sedation, and oxygen. The cause is generally neoplastic in developed countries, but more often tuberculous among poor and undernourished populations.

Impacted foreign bodies

See **Collapse and coma** and **Foreign bodies**

Children with respiratory emergencies always need assessment by an experienced paediatrician.

■ Rib fractures

See **Chest injuries**

■ Rings, finger

Casualty staff are experts with soap and water and persuasion. The nurses will show you how to remove tight rings with a ribbon. If that doesn't work, the ring-cutter is easy and effective. Rings should *always* be removed from injured or infected limbs.

■ Sheep tick

Holiday-makers suffer from this infestation more often than shepherds. It usually presents as a painless or slightly irritant pink purse, 0.5–1.0 cm in length, attached to the skin of the abdomen. The routine treatment is to press the blades of a fine curved artery forceps on the skin on either side of the thorax of the tick at the site of entry, spray the abdomen of the insect with ethyl chloride to induce it to let go, close the forceps, and avulse sharply. The removal is generally complete and the death and sterilization of any residue is ensured by painting twice daily with tincture of iodine for 3 days. Give tetanus toxoid antigen as required.

■ Shock, surgical (reduced circulating blood volume)

It is important when making your decision what to infuse, and how much, to consider the following basic questions:

What is the aim of infusion?

- Is it to save life now?
- Is it to render the patient fit for surgery after transfer elsewhere?
- Is it to gratify an irrational intravenous urge?

How much has the patient lost?

- Has he lost blood?
- Has he lost plasma?
- Is he still losing?

What does he need?

- Does he need simple fluid?
- Does he need plasma?
- Does he need blood volume?
- Does he need blood?

It is useless to pour anything into a bleeding patient when blood loss is continuing untreated. If blood loss cannot be staunched in the accident department intravenous infusion may keep him alive until he can reach the theatre for this to be done under general anaesthesia. But, if bleeding is severe, it may need to be done with O rhesus-negative blood or with plasma expanders (q.v.) before properly cross-matched blood is ready. If you work in a big unit which has its own theatres and a trauma surgeon, your patient has the best chance of recovery. In smaller units transfer from A & E to theatre often presents difficulties and delays, but it is of paramount importance to make it swiftly and effectively when the occasion demands. Try to use a micropore filter if you think that infusion of more than two units of blood is likely to be needed, because micro-aggregates in blood may damage the lungs; the need for rapid infusion may prevent its use. Give 10% calcium gluconate, 10 ml, if more than 4 units of blood are transfused. A blood-warmer is useful if rapid transfusion is required.

It is entirely useless, not to say positively harmful, to continue pouring non-haemoglobin-containing fluids into an exsanguinating patient, as the result is only to produce dilution of the blood that remains. A drop of 70% of circulating haemoglobin will be fatal in an acutely injured and bleeding patient who is otherwise healthy. Therefore give Haemaccel for urgent blood volume replacement unless the loss is of plasma (e.g. in extensive burning) and get blood *urgently* to continue the infusion until the

patient can be taken to theatre. If you use dextran, take the blood sample for cross-matching before starting the infusion; if you use Haemaccel no such precaution is required.

Cf. **'Plasma expanders'**

Patients in surgical shock who need analgesia should be given it intravenously in small doses, repeated as necessary. Intramuscular injections in shocked patients may not be appreciably absorbed owing to peripheral circulatory shutdown; when normal circulation is restored they will then exert a delayed, unwanted, and probably unrecognized effect.

Cf. **Pain**

Example

A patient with multiple injuries arrives in the accident department, having already lost 3 litres of blood from his circulating volume. Taking 6 litres as his estimated normal circulating volume, he has lost 50% of his haemoglobin (i.e. oxygen-carrying) complement. If you then infuse 3 litres of non-blood of any kind you will have effectively reduced his haemoglobin by a further 50%, i.e. to 25%. If his bleeding continues and infusion of non-blood is maintained the haemoglobin will rapidly fall to levels incompatible with cerebral survival.

Military antishock suit/trousers (MAST)   An original pneumatic tamponade device for the treatment of shock; not yet fully explored or validated, but popular in the USA as first aid. It consists of three segments, one for each leg and one for the pelvis and abdomen. It offers help in restoring central blood volume and controlling major pelvic bleeding in young victims of violent trauma, who often die of this. It does not replace blood transfusion.

Conclusion

Infusion of up to 2 litres of Haemaccel in the accident department is a first aid measure in the treatment of surgical shock. If more than this is required it is essential to give blood. If there is continuing blood loss which cannot be controlled, *instant transfer to the theatre is essential.*

■ Skin emergencies

These occur infrequently but skin conditions are sometimes presented to A & E units. They are best recognized from experience in a dermatological clinic or General Practitioner's surgery. Illustrated textbooks are helpful (see **Bibliography**) but verbal descriptions not. Once the condition is recognized the patient should be passed on to the appropriate person, dermatologist or General Practitioner.

True emergencies such as pemphigus and erythroderma seldom reach the A & E unit, but, if they do, need admission. They respond to parenteral steroids, but nearly always need nursing care and continuing supervision.

Surgical

Replacement of large ablations of *senile or steroid skins* caused by traffic, domestic, and horticultural calamities often gives unexpectedly successful results and saves much distress; it is always worth trying. Careful defatting of skin and debridement of the recipient area are essential; elevation is needed if a limb is involved.

Cf. **Injuries, minor**, pretibial lacerations, and **Grafts, skin**

Lumps and bumps

Many accident departments run a lumps and bumps service, as they are the best equipped to deal with them. They need out-patient treatment, patience, care, and follow-up. Keratoacanthomata, epitheliomata, basal cell carcinomata, naevi, various cysts, lipomata, fibromata, warts, and, alas, malignant melanomata all turn up from time to time. Any malignant or unusual skin conditions should be transferred for specialist opinion.

See also **Impetigo** and **Viruses**

■ Soft tissue injuries

Skin

Good skin repair using elementary plastic surgical techniques up to specialist standard should be the aim in A & E units. Remember that infantile skin has an almost infinite capacity for regeneration and repair; the tougher the skin the tougher the road to recovery. Heavy manual workers' skins can be slow and difficult to heal, needing prolonged and painstaking aftercare.

Muscle

Careful debridement is essential: make sure that all dead tissue is excised and all external contaminants removed and liberally washed out, using hydrogen peroxide; then suture carefully according to surgical principles. Provide adequate support or splintage in a relaxed position with early movement as the situation indicates. If serious injury demands splintage for the joints above and below the repair, energetic movement of more remote joints is to be insisted on so as to maintain circulation and venous return.

Tendons

See **Tendon injuries, miscellaneous** and **Tendon repairs, hand**

Nerves

For repair of digital nerves, see **Hand infections and injuries**.

Repair of major nerves (e.g. median or ulnar at the wrist or radial at the elbow or mid-arm) is a job for the highly specialized surgeon who is prepared to use micro-surgical techniques. If no such is available any experienced surgeon prepared to take pains must be found. This type of repair is in a 'growing region' of surgery and one must look forward to new advances all the time.

See also **Injuries, minor; Suture materials and techniques**, and **Wounds**

■ Stab wounds

These always need to be regarded with great suspicion. Three instances are given here of their latent dangers, and illustrate this point.

Stabs in the back

There may by an insignificant skin wound with no bleeding and the patient may complain of very little, but there may be a slowly accumulating haemothorax or haemopneumothorax which has no definite signs initially. All need chest X-ray and observation; a few need exploration.

Cf. **Chest injuries**

Stabs in the belly

The same caution applies. A negligible skin wound may be given by a small sharp instrument, and a probe may find no way through the sliding planes of the abdominal parietes, and yet there may be a small bowel perforation which could be fatal if it is unrecognized. An erect abdominal film may show air under the diaphragm, but even if it does not, admission for observation is essential, and exploration if there is any doubt about the extent of the injury.

Cf. **Abdominal injuries**

Stabs in the groin

Butchers boning beef can sustain lacerations of the femoral vein or its saphenous tributaries which become occluded by interstitial pressure for a few hours, only to break out again through normal walking movements disturbing the clot and altering local tissue relationships. Bleeding from this area can be rapid and severe. Careful exploration of the whole wound is obligatory.

Glass wounds should always be regarded as deeply penetrating until it is proved otherwise.

There are many variations on this theme (such as flying spicules of glass or metal) and they must always be borne in mind. A dramatic example of an unexpected outcome is afforded by the history of the little boy brought in with acute distress and cerebral disturbance, but with no external stigma apart from a tiny wound in his right upper eyelid. In the event it became clear that he had been playing in the garden with the broken blade of a miniature hacksaw, had fallen forwards on it in such a way that it passed through the orbit (missing the eye), through the superior orbital fissure and into the brain, penetrating as far back as the thalamus on the same side. He died about 10 hours later after coma, fits, and hyperthermia. The blade was found later in the garden with his blood on it. He must have pulled it out himself an instant after wounding.

■ Stings, etc. by marine creatures

Stinging creatures in the sea can cause death, especially amongst children in tropical waters. If early treatment can be given with intravenous antihistamines and topical and systemic steroids, and in anaphylactoid types of reaction with intramuscular adrenaline, lives can be saved. General supportive treatment is needed as well.

Cf. **Stings, wasp and bee** and **Anaphylaxis, acute**

Examples of stinging creatures are jellyfish (e.g. *Aurelia aurita*) and the dangerous Mediterranean *Physalia* (Portuguese man-of-war), weaver fish, sting ray, and other stingers in tropical waters. The unfriendly habit of Mediterranean sea urchins of leaving their spines in bathers' soles is well known. These produce an intensely painful foreign body reaction and, even after careful removal, a persistent area of sensitivity and inflammation which may need topical steroid treatment, with occlusion, to obtain relief. The reaction can last for some months. Immediate soaking in acetone is said to dissolve the spines. Jamaican fishermen recommend rum.

■ Stings, wasp and bee

A vast number of people attends A & E departments annually for this tiresome affliction. It is simplest to issue a 3-day course of chlorpheniramine (Piriton) tablets, 4 mg thrice daily, as a routine. But a few come who suffer from severe local or general reactions. These need intramuscular or intravenous chlorpheniramine 10 mg at once, and a 3-day course of tablets. Patients who show anaphylactic reactions with tachycardia and collapse need intramuscular adrenaline, and occasionally intravenous fluids and admission. Intravenous hydrocortisone 100 mg is worthwhile in severely collapsed cases.

Cf. **Anaphylaxis, acute**

These patients should always receive a course of desensitizing injections against wasp or bee venom because anaphylactic reactions may put the victim's life in jeopardy, and wasp and bee venom hyposensitization is effective: Pharmalgen wasp venom and Pharmalgen bee venom are available from Pharmacia Diagnostics. They need to be given in a hospital environment, at least to start with, under observation by an experienced person able to deal with the earliest signs of anaphylaxis. Not to give them when a patient has experienced an anaphylactic reaction is hardly justifiable.

■ Stridor, acute

Acute stridor in a young child may be due to:

Acute viral croup usually follows 2 or 3 days of upper respiratory tract infection and the child is afebrile and exhibits stridor only when upset. There is always a barking cough. Intubation is rarely needed but the child may become cyanosed or exhausted, with stridor at rest. Admit.

Acute epiglottitis usually follows upper respiratory symptoms of less than 24 hours duration and there is obvious toxaemia; the child may be febrile and drools his secretions and has severe stridor; coughing is rare. Complete airway obstruction may develop within minutes. Procedures that can cause crying, *including examination of the throat*, can precipitate laryngeal obstruction and should wait until a stable airway has been established by intubation by an *experienced* anaesthetist, if epiglottitis is suspected (Tarnow-Mordi, W. O., Berrill, A. M., Darby, C. W., Davis, P., and Pook, J. (1985). Precipitation of laryngeal obstruction in acute epiglottitis. *British Medical Journal*, **290**, 629). Do not sedate the child, although he is very restless. A lateral X-ray of the neck may be requested to confirm the diagnosis but there is not universal agreement about its value; certainly it must not be allowed to interfere with the progress of

treatment. Most children with epiglottitis require intubation; *Haemophilus influenzae* is the usual culprit and may be resistant to ampicillin, so that intravenous chloramphenicol is needed. Steroids may possibly help. In very urgent cases, laryngostomy (q.v.) may be life-saving. Acute epiglottitis must be dealt with by senior doctors throughout its management.

Staphylococcal laryngotracheobronchitis shares the clinical features of both viral croup and acute epiglottitis but leads to the production of copious thick secretions. Intubation is needed, and frequent tracheal aspiration.

Foreign body inhalation is often heralded by an attack of coughing. See **Foreign bodies**.

Angio-oedema is often but not always associated with soft tissue swelling elsewhere.

The widely accepted clinical features which differentiate acute viral croup from epiglottitis are not totally reliable (Milner, A. D. (1984). Acute stridor in the preschool child. *British Medical Journal,* **288**, 811–12).

Any child at risk of upper airway obstruction should be given oxygen; he may require very urgent intubation, which can be exceptionally difficult, and he must be admitted and seen by an experienced paediatrician urgently. Consultation with an ENT surgeon and an anaesthetist is often required.

■ Suicide, attempted

This is no longer a crime but is usually a demonstration of withdrawal from an emotionally intolerable situation or a demand for attention rather than a determined attempt to 'end it all'. Every case should be seen by a psychiatrist before leaving hospital.

See **Psychiatric emergencies**

Attempted suicides among children under 14 (especially boys) and adults over 60 (especially men) are often serious attempts. The children, from deep affection, feel

that the other treatments are no good or obnoxious is
unacceptable but often, less trenchantly, disagree or
always more in interpretation are so in effect that they
cannot be?

Suture materials and techniques

The choice of suture materials is difficult to resolve with as
many answers as there are clinicians. Sutures in use can be
subdivided as follows:

- Suture material to absorb.
- Suture material non-reactive, etc.
- Rate about which a suture is, etc.

In addition to the above you have to consider the
strength and elasticity, the diameter of the material and
also the choice of the needle (range of reaction needed)
when suturing will obtain. To complicate matters, overall
precautions present much depends on the type of
which the wound is at. In the situation of obvious all are
not always in danger.

The needle best, the perfect suture, material or suture?
The advantage of absorbed material is that it is generally
easier with the accomplishment of dead reaction of its
reduction of friction, there is which on fracture, thus
protecting the change of the amount of suture needed
to arrive during its course. Be too even the absorbable
discard suture that you use too much through tissue
than absorbable, etc. the resulting may can cause
tissue trauma.

For tissue muscle it is wise to bear in the more
absorbent and dissolvable material should remain ideally (a)
repaired shortly is advised.

Minimum is the weaker the level, requirements for
muscle and particularly the faster site such of the material
more satisfactory a needle that be used also at situation
required forces which case the amount of suture needed
with the minimum risk as required into the tissue.

The delicate and surgical the amount is that the more
nervous tissue, the nerves that are would be special for

that life after their parents are divorced or separated is intolerable; the elderly, from loneliness, despair, or disease, make the determined effort to be rid of what they cannot bear.

■ Suture materials and techniques

The choice of these presents a difficult problem with as many answers as practitioners. Suture materials can be subdivided as follows:

- Source: natural or synthetic
- Structure: monofilament or braided
- Fate: absorbable or non-absorbable

In addition to the above, you have to consider the strength (and therefore the thickness) of a material, and also the design of the needle (cutting or round-bodied) when making your choice. To complicate matters even further, the eventual result depends upon the time for which the suture is left in the wound and, above all, the dexterity of the surgeon.

The search for the perfect suture material continues. The advantage of braided material is that it is generally easier to tie than monofilament; its disadvantage lies in its tendency to harbour bacteria within its structure, thus increasing the chances of infection. Certainly braided material (e.g. silk) must not be used with abscesses (q.v.). Braided sutures tend to pass less easily through tissue than monofilaments and the resulting drag can cause tissue trauma.

For facial wounds it is wisest to use a fine non-absorbable monofilament material and remove it early (at about 4 days) if possible.

Material to be left within the body (e.g. deep sutures to muscle) is generally absorbable (e.g. catgut or Dexon) but non-absorbable material can be used (e.g. for tendon repairs). Lacerations inside the mouth are best sutured with absorbable material, as removal can be difficult.

The thicker the material, the stronger it is, but the more obvious is the final scar. 2/0 or 3/0 would be typical for

the thigh or knee; about 3/0 for the trunk and 4/0 for the arm; 5/0 for an adult's face; 6/0 for a child's face, or even 7/0 if the eyelid is involved. Clearly these are approximations and each case must be taken on its merits.

In general, the thicker the material used, the longer it is left in: again because a strong repair is needed. Three or 4 days is adequate for the face; 6 or 7 days for the arms or trunk; 9 or 10 days for the lower limbs. The longer the material remains in place, the more obvious the scar; however the fine monofilament synthetic sutures can be left for surprisingly long periods with minimal reaction.

Interrupted sutures tend to be used more often than continuous in A & E units, because of the relatively dirty nature of the wounds compared to the sterile wounds made by surgeons in theatre: if infection does develop, one or two sutures can be removed, whereas the entire wound would have to be laid open if the suturing was continuous. It doesn't matter whether you tie your knots with your hands or with instruments, as long as they fall flat and bring the skin edges neatly together without overlap. Take as small a bite as you are able without running the risk of the stitch cutting out. A few key sutures, strategically placed at the onset, often make accurate apposition easier, with a consequently neater final result.

■ Tendon injuries, miscellaneous

Ruptured biceps (long head)

See **Injuries, minor**

Abductor pollicis longus + extensor pollicis longus

Whether divided singly or together, these need surgical repair in working men. In elderly women after Colles' fractures, rupture of extensor pollicis longus may be best left alone; some repair it; seek orthopaedic advice.

Quadriceps femoris tendon (supra- and infra-patellar)

Rupture is often associated with injury to the joint capsule. This is very much an orthopaedic problem.

Achilles tendon

Rupture is historically characterized by the feeling as of a blow on the calf or below it, while running or jumping, and is usually accompanied by a fall. Most orthopaedic surgeons prefer primary repair followed by an equinus plaster. Admit.

Cf. **Injuries, minor**, Ruptured plantaris tendon

■ Tendon repairs, hand

The primary concern of a casualty officer dealing with a potential tendon injury in the hand is *recognition*. These injuries are often missed and their diagnosis is described in detail in **Hand infections and injuries**.

Extensor tendons

There is little disagreement about the primary repair of extensor tendons in the A & E department. They rarely retract and repair should be a routine procedure in which all senior and some junior staff are proficient. The conditions provided should be of operating theatre standard, as far as it is possible to achieve this in A & E circumstances, and the steps are approximately as follows:

1 Extensive skin preparation.
2 Scrupulous cleaning and debridement of skin wounds with careful assessment of available skin flaps. Mobilization of existing flaps gives much more effective skin cover and should be done whenever feasible; grafting is a last resort, but better than no skin.

3   Dissection of both ends of a completely divided tendon for at least 1 cm above and below the division. Where the tendon is expanded it should be sutured with interrupted 3/0 or 4/0 prolene stitches. Where the tendon is cylindrical an initial stitch (Kleinert's method preferred: see Fig. 9) using a suture with a needle on both ends is required, and interrupted stitches afterwards. This gives a secure hold without cutting through the tendon.

4   Skin closure with 4/0 prolene, carried out with the greatest attention to detail in obtaining good apposition while preserving blood supply.

5   Minimum dressing applied.

6   Minimal but logical extension splintage, to keep all tension off the suture line. Thus if the injury is (a) on the dorsum of the hand or at the metacarpophalangeal joint, the wrist should be fixed in extension with plaster of Paris from the lower third of the forearm to the distal phalanx; (b) distal to the metacarpophalangeal joint and proximal to the distal interphalangeal joint, Zimmer splintage (padded, malleable aluminium strip) from proximal to the metacarpophalangeal joint to distal to the distal interphalangeal joint; (c) distal to (b), splint from finger tip to middle of proximal phalanx. Splints should be as small as is possible to do the job, so as to allow as much movement as possible without putting stress on the suture line. Splintage is required for about 3 weeks, and is followed by gentle, active mobilization. The results are good, often better than you would think possible.

In complicated, multiple, or comminuted injuries of the hand and fingers, when all possible repairing has been done, a volar slab gives the best support. It should extend from elbow to finger tips, ideally with the metacarpophalangeal joints at 90° and the interphalangeal joints extended (see Fig. 10).

Mallet finger: see **Fractures, hand.**

Boutonnière deformity   This is due to rupture of the central slip of the extensor expansion, which is inserted

into the base of the middle phalanx. First, the remnants, before reattachment, are passed through a proximal interphalangeal slip and ... over ... the digital ... ... position. This is ... reduce the profundal insertion ... loose attachment ... ... means to ... an open ... ... tendon and then suture the ... ...

Flexor tendons

All lacerated flexor tendons must be recognised at first attendance. ... should both ends and retained and explored in the hands theatre of a plastic surgeon immediately ... ... as a primary repair. They should not be repaired ... ... extensive.

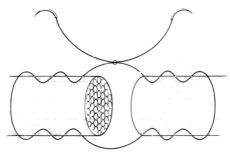

Fig. 9.

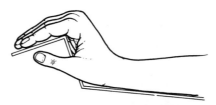

Fig. 10. Volar slab plaster of Paris for extensor tendon injuries and hand fractures (especially metacarpal and proximal phalanx). Metacarpophalangeal joint at 90°; wrist joint at 60°.

into the base of the middle phalanx; the resultant deformity consists of flexion of the proximal interphalangeal joint and hyperextension of the distal interphalangeal joint. For a closed injury, the proximal interphalangeal joint should be splinted in extension for 6 weeks; for an open division, repair the tendon and then splint the joint.

Flexor tendons

All flexor tendon injuries must be diagnosed at first attendance (see **Hand infections and injuries**) and referred to an orthopaedic surgeon or a plastic surgeon immediately, with a view to primary repair. They should *not* be repaired by a casualty officer.

■ Tenosynovitis and tenovaginitis

Tenosynovitis is a common cause of pain in the forearm, often with swelling over the affected tendons (most often the extensors of the thumb and the radial extensors of the wrist). It frequently follows repetitive over-use and can occur in any long tendons with tendon sheaths. Crepitus is common but not constant. Treatment is with plaster of Paris for 10 days to 3 weeks, according to the severity; concurrent anti-inflammatory drugs should be used. Give an injection of lignocaine and methylprednisolone (Depo-Medrone) 40 mg if plaster of Paris is not successful; this is not the ideal primary treatment as it has its own perils and may lead to too early reuse of the affected limb, with obstinate recurrence of the disorder; I prefer to use it as a secondary remedy. Remember to apply the plaster with due regard to effective immobilization of the affected tendon; a Colles' type of plaster, for example, is of no use to immobilize an inflamed extensor pollicis longus tendon.

Suppurative tenosynovitis

See **Hand infections and injuries**

de Quervain's tenovaginitis stenosans involves the tendons of extensor pollicis brevis and/or abductor pollicis longus, in the fibro-osseous canal at the radial styloid. There is pain, tenderness, and a palpable nodule. It is commonest in middle-aged women. Passive adduction of the wrist or thumb causes pain. The canal frequently has to be surgically explored and laid open, with uniformly successful results.

Tenovaginitis stenosans of the flexor pollicis longus tendon at the metacarpophalangeal joint presents in little boys (usually under 4 years old) as a fixed flexion deformity at the interphalangeal joint of the thumb; it is often bilateral and the tender nodule responsible for it is palpable at the metacarpophalangeal joint. This condition is responsive to surgery, though in babies it is worth waiting a few months as spontaneous recovery may occur.

In middle-aged women it generally presents as a painful, clicking, sometimes briefly locking, abnormality of finger or thumb flexion; when the clenched hand is unclenched, the digit remains flexed and may suddenly straighten with a snap ('triggering') or may require passive extension, again with a snap; a tender nodule is palpable anterior to the metacarpophalangeal joint. Again surgery is required. Local anaesthesia allows the active co-operation of the patient and assures adequate release of the constriction.

■ Tetanus prophylaxis

Tetanus is a fearful disease which can be prevented by immunization. **Active immunity** is preferable. An intramuscular injection of 0.5 ml of adsorbed tetanus toxoid (ATT), followed by a second after 6 weeks, and a third after 6 months, will build up sufficient immunity to overcome potential infection. Thereafter, a booster dose is required every 5 years; such a booster will result in a rapid rise of antibody levels.

In practice, therefore, a patient with a laceration (and remember that any laceration, however small, is a potential source of tetanus) can be placed in one of the following categories:

- Full course within the last 5 years
  Action: reassurance
- Full course more than 5 years ago; booster dose in last 5 years
  Action: reassurance
- Full course more than 5 years ago; no booster dose in last 5 years
  Action: booster dose of ATT
- Course begun at some stage but never completed
  Action: booster dose of ATT and refer to own GP for second and third injections at 6 weeks and 6 months

- Never had any prophylaxis
  Action: give first injection of ATT and refer to own GP for second and third injections at 6 weeks and 6 months
- Immune status unknown
  Action: booster dose of ATT and refer to own GP (who will have records) for further action as necessary.

A patient who has sustained a very dirty and contused wound (unless it is absolutely certain that he has had a full course of immunization at some stage, with booster doses at 5 yearly intervals) should be given **passive immunity** with human immunoglobulin (Humotet), 1 ml, *as well as* active immunity with ATT. The Humotet and the ATT should be given at separate sites. The passive immunity provided by the Humotet will tide the patient over the time during which he is developing active immunity from the ATT.

Remember, though, that neither ATT nor Humotet are substitutes for thorough cleansing and debridement of the wound.

Parents sometimes arrive with children who have never been immunized. This may be due to parental apathy ('I never bothered') or parental ignorance ('I don't agree with his having injections', implying that they do agree with his having tetanus). Equally common is for parents (both father and mother) to be unaware whether their child has ever had any injections. We have travelled so far along the path of the welfare state that all personal and parental and filial responsibilities have been abandoned by many.

The only rational policy in an A & E unit is to aim at universal immunization. Every patient attending should be offered immunization; every injured patient should be recommended to accept it, unless known to be allergic to ATT. Documentation should be universal and thorough.

■ Thoracic intubation

In cases of chest injury in which you suspect tension pneumothorax or haemo(pneumo)thorax, intercostal intubation may be life-saving in the early stages of reception.

Identify a tension pneumothorax by passing a hollow needle between the second and third ribs in the mid-clavicular line. If air audibly escapes, intubate and connect the cannula to an underwater seal or one-way valve system. If common sense, examination, and radiography suggest that there is an accumulating haemothorax, intubation will materially assist pulmonary expansion, and so cerebral oxygenation, in addition to giving a useful indication of intrathoracic blood loss.

Intubation is best done with a trocar-mounted cannula. Under local anaesthesia, the skin and underlying tissues should be incised down to the parietal pleura by means of a scalpel cut 2 cm in length (in the intercostal space just above the rib below) before inserting the trocar and cannula. The apparatus should be grasped in the gloved hand like a dagger held 5 cm from its tip: this will avoid too deep a penetration. Rapid attachment to a previously prepared underwater seal follows. The cannula can then be gently passed into the chest for a convenient distance and anchored to the skin with a stitch. Apply a waterproof dressing and check the position of the cannula with a chest X-ray. If you use an axillary or posterior approach you run the risk of perforating the liver, spleen, or bowel which has wandered into the chest through a tear in the diaphragm.

Cf. **Chest injuries** and **Pneumothorax**

Torticollis, acute

This is characterized by onset at night. The young patient wakes with a painful wry neck: one of the sternocleido-mastoid muscles is in spasm and the head is turned to the opposite side. X-ray is not needed. It can also occur during exertion and is common in the winter, less common in the summer. X-ray is advisable in patients over 25 years old. It is distinguished from cervical prolapsed intervertebral disc by the absence of root signs, and by the age group.

Treatment

Spray the skin over the painful area with local pain-relieving spray, such as ethyl chloride, and apply slow, forced rotation to the neutral position; apply a soft collar. Cure within 48 hours is usual, within 24 hours likely, within one hour frequent. Give analgesics if necessary. Very severe cases may need general anaesthesia.

Cf. **Necks**

Tracheostomy

Tracheostomy should never be undertaken as an emergency procedure, for the following reasons:

- It is not easy to do, if it is to be done properly, as the trachea is a long way from the skin at the desirable level
- Properly placed tracheostomy involves division of the thyroid isthmus, and in an asphyxiated patient the inevitable bleeding is likely to lead to contamination of the airway at least, and blockage of the trachea at most
- Improperly placed tracheostomy is likely to need refashioning (with all the attendant complications) if required for a long time. If it is not wanted for more than a day or so the operation is unnecessary
- It takes too long to meet an emergency

Therefore in cases of asphyxia which cannot be overcome by intubation, **laryngostomy** (q.v.) is the emergency operation of choice.

■ Tuberculosis

Three presentations can occur as emergencies:

Acute pulmonary (miliary tuberculosis)

This is not a cachectic presentation but a subacute bronchopneumonia with fever and characteristic radiological features.

Glandular

This is not uncommon in cervical glands in children, presenting as single, or groups of, rubbery glands and diagnosed by excision biopsies. In the elderly it presents as chronic, caseating, cervical abscesses.

Bone and joint tuberculosis

This is common in immigrants to the United Kingdom. Spinal cases present with backache, malaise, and loss of weight. There are other bone and joint manifestations. Early identification is very important. It is also common in poor or malnourished communities world-wide.

■ Ulcers, gravitational

The chronic ulcers which used to provide material for a weekly clinic in many casualty departments of the past were more remarkable for their foul smell than for the effectiveness of any remedy supplied. Mercifully they exist no more and should never return, because of an improved understanding of the role of compression treatment of gravitational ischaemia. In the acute phase they should be treated with sterile foam pads soaked in an

antiseptic solution (e.g. povidone-iodine 10% in water), kept in position by elastic bandages or Tubigrip and encouraged by regular walking exercise and strict elevation when sitting. These need changing every 2 or 3 days until infection is controlled and healing has begun. Then they should be replaced by weekly application of Ichthopaste bandages expertly applied (see **Bandages**) until the ulcers are healed. Then it must be made clear that appropriate elastic support is essential for evermore unless surgery (e.g. varicose vein stripping) can remedy the underlying cause.

If you meet an ulcer which does not respond to this approach it may be that arterial ischaemia is responsible, or else that you ought to have done serological tests for syphilis: tertiary syphilis can still occur. Consider also the possibility of squamous cell carcinoma or artefact injury.

There is a wide variety of local applications available for controlling infection and hastening epithelialization. Ensuring adequate venous return is the basic and permanent need.

■ Unconsciousness

Common causes

- Self-poisoning: history and absence of physical signs (see **Poisoning**)
- Cerebrovascular accident (see **Neurological emergencies**)
- Epilepsy: history and scars (see **Collapse and coma** and **Confusion, acute**)
- Diabetes: instant diagnosis with Dextrostix (see **Diabetic emergencies**)
- Cardiovascular collapse (see **Cardiac arrest** and **Cardiovascular emergencies, other**)
- Febrile convulsions: see **Convulsions, febrile**
- Trauma: usually self-evident, but often associated with an alcoholic component (see **Drunkenness**)

Rare causes

Miscellaneous, such as:

- Uraemia: see **Collapse and coma**
- Addisonian crisis: see **Endocrine emergencies**
- Anaphylactic shock (see **Anaphylaxis, acute**): note especially wasp stings (see **Stings, wasp and bee**)
- Waterhouse–Friderichsen syndrome and various others too rare to merit inclusion (see **Collapse and coma**)

Cf. **Collapse and coma**

■ Urogenital emergencies

Anuria

Primary anuria is a medical emergency unlikely to arise in the A & E department; secondary anuria can be due to hypovolaemic shock (see **Shock, surgical**) or to the crush syndrome. The latter syndrome was identified in the First World War, forgotten, re-identified in the Second World War, and forgotten again until the Moorgate tube train disaster in February 1975, when it made itself remembered again. It should never be forgotten; it is caused by the blockage of renal tubules by products of myoglobin breakdown, which follows the release of the circulatory return from areas of prolonged muscle ischaemia, such as that due to crushing entrapment of a limb. It is the *only* condition which requires a tourniquet as first aid treatment and emergency amputation as the definitive treatment. It should not be confused with renal shutdown.

Cf. **Urogenital injuries**

Balanitis

This can produce acute urinary retention and normally responds to frequent hot baths, and antibiotic eye-ointment applied inside the prepuce. In urgent cases a dorsal slit may be required: easily performed under lignocaine 1%. The subsequent need for formal circumcision should not be forgotten, and careful follow-up is important. Fungal balanitis also occurs but is seldom acute.

Colic, renal

This is familiar to every house officer and may be accompanied by haematuria. It is a common entrée for drug addicts as it is easily simulated and difficult to disprove. Abdominal X-ray may show a stone.

Epididymo-orchitis

This should never be diagnosed in young men except in the presence of active urinary or venereal infection; likewise orchitis should never be diagnosed in anyone at all except in the presence of mumps. In young men and boys every such case is a testicular torsion unless proved otherwise, that is by operation.

Gynaecological emergencies (q.v.)

Haematospermia

This is not uncommon in young men and generally of no import. It can accompany new growths such as seminoma testis, but is a late sign.

Haematuria

This may be associated with great fear but seldom requires urgent treatment. Investigation requires admission.

Oliguria

As a complication of injury is a manifestation of hypo-volaemic shock. Every victim of major or multiple injuries should be catheterized (with an indwelling balloon catheter) and the output monitored as a routine.

Paraphimosis

This must be reduced even if there is not urethral occlusion, as swelling can occur rapidly. The standard textbook reduction by two thumbs is often effective after intravenous midazolam (see **Dislocations**). If this is unsuccessful a dorsal slit should be performed with blunt-ended scissors after infiltration with lignocaine. In children, general anaesthesia is needed. The dorsal slit operation is safer, more effective, and less liable to recurrence than the standard operation of dividing the compressing ring. Subsequent elective circumcision may be needed to tidy up unsightly flaps.

Phimosis

This seldom produces total retention. Formal circumcision as an emergency or elective procedure is better than stretching. In the aged a dorsal slit may be kinder and as effective.

Retention of urine

Acute retention is agonizing and needs early relief by catheterization. Always use a balloon type of self-retaining catheter, leave it in place attached to a urine bag, and admit the patient for observation. Local urethral analgesia with lignocaine gel 2% is a source of comfort to the patient and makes catheterization more uniformly successful. If catheterization is impossible, dilatation of a stricture may be needed, using urethral bougies; this needs practice, but the art can be acquired readily. In remote areas every doctor dealing with emergencies should be able to cope. Receiving surgeons fall into four

classes: those who say 'How dare you lay your filthy hands on my patients?' (reply: 'To relieve their pain.'); those who say 'Why don't you put in a catheter instead of bothering me?' (reply: 'To avoid the first response.'); and those who use both gambits alternately; there is a small class who respond rationally and they should be cultivated as assiduously as a vegetable garden in a famine.

Chronic retention with overflow is best decompressed in stages so as to avoid reactive bleeding from the kidneys and bladder wall. Some urologists like to do this themselves after admission, but if pain is severe it is not kind to delay.

Regular catheterization of paraplegics sometimes falls to the lot of A & E staff. Every 3 or 4 weeks is optimum and silicone-coated catheters are best.

Stone in the bladder

Seldom a source of emergency, but it can present as severe intermittent pain related to posture and can interfere with micturition. It is commoner in men than in women, in hot dry climates than in temperate, in poor communities than in rich.

Testicular torsion

Never diagnose orchitis in young men and boys except in the presence of mumps. A tender or painful testis must always be regarded as due to torsion until proved otherwise. This is a surgical emergency which is too often missed. It may resolve spontaneously but in a high proportion of untreated cases the poor patient is left with one ineffective gonad. Every case should be referred to a surgeon urgently.

Venereal disease (q.v.)

See also **Urogenital injuries**

■ Urogenital injuries

Renal injury

Renal injury usually presents with haematuria and/or loin pain. There may be signs of severe internal bleeding and serial clinical and radiological examination may reveal an enlarging haematoma in the loin. An intravenous urogram may show damage and will also demonstrate the function of the opposite kidney. Most renal injuries settle with bed rest and repeated observations but exploration is sometimes required.

Injury to the bladder

Intraperitoneal rupture presents with severe shock and peritonism: urgent exploration is required. Extraperitoneal rupture is almost always associated with a fractured pelvis: again immediate surgery is necessary.

Urethral injury, suspected

It is very important to look for this injury, especially in young male victims of pelvic fractures from road traffic accidents or from being rolled on by their fallen horses. Difficulty in passing urine and urethral bleeding are the presenting symptoms. Severe urethral injuries are often associated with severe blood loss and perineal bruising. Urological surgeons vary in their approach and you have to know what your own specialist prefers. If catheterization is required it should be done very gently with a fine, soft catheter and only on direct instruction by the surgeon consulted; you must avoid converting a partial rupture of the urethra into a complete rupture, increasing bleeding, or making a false passage. If one gentle attempt at catheterization is unsuccessful, a suprapubic catheter may be needed. Some surgeons prefer to have a urethrogram done as a primary procedure.

■ Venereal disease

1 Take a plain swab into trichomonas transport medium.
2 Take a charcoal swab into Stuart's transport medium.
3 Take blood for syphilis serology and gonococcal fixation test ('VD serology' is a safe omnibus request).
4 Make dry slides for Gram-staining.
5 Send all 4 urgently to the laboratory.
6 Refer the patient to the next genito-urinary medicine clinic at the appropriate time and place; he/she must abstain from sexual intercourse in the interim.
7 Advise the patient that his/her partner(s) will also need treatment.

Genital herpes: refer for identification and treatment in all cases. Cf. **Viruses.**

Acquired immune deficiency syndrome (AIDS) is a new and frightening disease; zidovudine may be of benefit. Keep abreast of developments. Refer to the local expert.

■ Violence

Unfortunately an increasing source of injuries and of management problems in accident units. General violence (varieties of mob hysteria and riot) is common and produces a wide variety of injuries; individual violence, often associated with drunkenness (q.v.), is commoner still at dances and outside pubs at closing time. The currently accepted form (1987) is for drunken idiot A to knock down drunken idiot B who is incapable of rising to retaliate; then A kicks B repeatedly in the face and trunk. Maxillo-facial injuries are common and often severe. Associated skin wounds are usually contused and difficult to repair.

This is a great and growing social problem in the West, reflected at all levels of society with varying degrees of sophistication; it is still chiefly verbal at the professional level.

Management of violent patients leans heavily for help on the police, who are very good at coping. This is another reason for maintaining good relationships with the force, within the bounds of confidentiality.

■ Viruses

Acute viral infections often arrive in the A & E department because symptoms may come suddenly and manifestations may be unfamiliar or confusing, and attributed to trauma. The briefest survey is all that is required here.

Herpes simplex (*labial* [cold sore]; *digital* [herpetic whitlow]; *genital*) is effectively treated with acyclovir; the earlier it is used, the greater the chance of success.

Herpes simplex keratitis (dendritic ulcer) is treated with acyclovir ophthalmic ointment, but needs urgent ophthalmological supervision.

Herpes zoster (shingles) presents with pain, followed a few days later by the characteristic rash stopping in the midline. Local lesions respond to acyclovir and an attack diagnosed early can often be aborted similarly. In the elderly, in whom post-herpetic neuralgia is such a dire consequence, the opportunity is never to be missed.

Herpes zoster ophthalmicus again needs expert ophthalmological supervision.

Bell's palsy may be due to a herpetic virus. Oral prednisolone (60 mg daily for 5 days, then 50 mg, 40 mg, 30 mg, 20 mg, 10 mg, and 5 mg on consecutive days) may help. The condition is probably of varied origin, so a variable response is to be expected.

Paravaccinia (milker's nodule) is generally a digital and uncomfortable lump. It is differentiated form orf by a history of contact with the relevant host. Its onset is fairly rapid and acyclovir may help.

Orf is a virus infection of the facial skin of sheep, occasionally transmitted to shepherds and children. Its appearance is characteristically that of a small, *painless* carbuncle, of slow onset. Secondary infection is generally a presenting symptom, possibly with lymphangitis and lymphadenopathy. Treatment is by antibiotics for the secondary infection and acyclovir for the primary lesion. It is slow to develop and fairly slow to go. Most commonly it occurs on the hand. *Erythema multiforme* is a common complication which merits a short course of oral steroids; it can be very severe and distressing.

Idoxuridine is an alternative antiviral agent to acyclovir.

See also **Venereal disease**

▆ Wounds

The general care of wounds is extremely important and not always sufficiently emphasized. An A & E department with a bad record of sepsis is one in which there is not a high enough standard of wound care. Antibiotics and antiseptics are not good substitutes.

Finger wounds should be cleaned to the wrist, hand wounds to the elbow, forearm wounds to the shoulder (above and below), and so on. Skin edges should be trimmed to make them neat and straight; remove epidermal tags, any devitalized tissue, and all visible foreign bodies; irrigate invisible foreign bodies with detergent solutions (e.g. cetrimide 1%) or with 6% hydrogen peroxide solution, remove grease with detergent jelly (e.g. Swarfega), dry the wound carefully, and only then repair. You cannot take too great pains at this task.

Suture should be carried out carefully and thoroughly so as to secure perfect apposition of skin edges without slackness, irregularity, or tension. The minimum of dressing and the maximum of ventilation is required. The wound will then be painless, clean, and quick to heal in ninety-nine cases out of a hundred. If primary closure is not possible, admission for subsequent grafting should be considered. Every hand wound should have a sling for 48 hours at least. Aftercare of skin wounds after healing (by application of surgical spirit after washing, or chlorhexidine cream to scabby wounds) reduces secondary infection to vanishing point.

Antibiotic sprays should never be used: they fill the air with allergogenic dust, and the department with multi-resistant bacteria. Povidone-iodine spray (Betadine) is a useful antiseptic application.

If you are making the wound yourself never forget that the skin you mean to cut must always be cleaned with a detergent first (soap and water or cetrimide 1%), dried, and then well painted with tincture of iodine (weak solution of iodine in spirit BP). Sensitivity to this preparation is rare, and reversible with steroid creams.

See also **Injuries, minor; Soft tissue injuries; Suture materials and techniques**

■ Wrist and hand amputations

Wrist and hand amputations and wounds involving the main nerves, tendons, and blood vessels are of increasing importance as specialist techniques for dealing with them improve. The use of microsurgical repair and its application to replantation operations offer new hope in these dreaded injuries.

If it is decided to refer a patient to a plastic surgeon for this type of operation, the detached finger or hand should be wrapped in sterile towels and enclosed in a thermostable container holding ice, but not allowed direct contact with it. Only clean-cut wounds are likely to be amenable to this treatment (e.g. guillotine amputations).

The longest possible warning should be given to the receiving unit as advance notice of an impending emergency operation which may take from 12 to 18 hours is obviously needed.

Cf. **Hand infections and injuries**

■ X-rays

These are dangerous and expensive. Requests for examinations and films should be limited and specific: 'shipping orders' strongly suggest that you haven't examined the patient adequately. Never ask for an X-ray without detailed examination and then make a specific request. For example if you suspect a fractured scaphoid it is useless to ask for 'X-ray of wrist', as the views will not be adequate. A fractured scaphoid often eludes primary detection; if it is suspected the radiographer, if requested, can perform special views (coned and oblique) to demonstrate the scaphoid, thus raising the frequency of primary diagnosis dramatically.

Cf. **Radiographers**

■ Zip-fastener calamities

Not uncommonly unfortunates present themselves with penile skin caught in the zip of their trousers, usually a fold of foreskin which is trapped in the slide. This can be rectified by destruction of the zip mechanism with a small pair of strong wire-cutters. A little local lignocaine 1% injected at the base of the involved fold of skin makes it easier for patient and casualty officer alike. It is rare for any suturing or other surgical work to be needed thereafter.

Bibliography

Apley, A. G. and Solomon, L. (1982). *System of ortho-paedics and fractures*, (6th edn). Butterworth, London. Short, complete, and clear.

Approved products for farmers and growers (1986). Issued by the Ministry of Agriculture, Fisheries and Food, HMSO.

Association of the British Pharmaceutical Industry (1986). *ABPI data sheet compendium*. Datapharm Publications, London. Updated regularly; invaluable.

Bache, J. B., Armitt, C. R., and Tobiss, J. R. (1985). *A colour atlas of nursing procedures in accidents and emergencies*. Wolfe Medical Publications, London. Full of practical procedures which the junior doctor must be able to perform; lavishly illustrated.

British national formulary. British Medical Association and The Pharmaceutical Society of Great Britain, London. Very good indeed; updated regularly.

Bron, A. J. (1983). *The unquiet eye: a diagnostic guide*. Glaxo Laboratories Ltd, Greenford.

Clain, A. (ed.) (1986). *Hamilton Bailey's demonstrations of physical signs in clinical surgery*, (17th edn). Wright, Bristol.

Conolly, W. B. and Kilgore, E. S. (1979). *Hand injuries and infections: an illustrated guide*. Edward Arnold, London.

Evans, T. R. (ed.) (1986). *ABC of resuscitation. British Medical Journal*, London.

Frohne, D. and Pfänder, H. J. (1984). *A colour atlas of poisonous plants*. Wolfe Medical Publications, London. An authoritative guide with good illustrations; comprehensive and reliable.

Fry, L. (1984). *Dermatology: an illustrated guide*, (3rd edn). Butterworth, London.

Gosselin, R. (ed.) (1984). *Clinical toxicology of commercial products*, (5th edn). Williams and Wilkins, London. The only available source book; very extensive and very useful but needs practice in use because of its American provenance and complicated layout; like all source books it is out of date after a year or so;

many limitations, especially cost and transatlantic nomenclature.

Grech, P. (1981). *Casualty radiology: a practical guide for radiological diagnosis.* Chapman and Hall, London.

Hope, R. A. and Longmore, J. M. (1985). *Oxford handbook of clinical medicine.* Oxford University Press. An excellent little book, which will fit into the pocket and contains a chapter devoted to emergencies.

Illingworth, C. M. (1982). *The diagnosis and primary care of accidents and emergencies in children,* (2nd edn). Blackwell Scientific Publications, Oxford. Unique.

Jackson, R. H. (1977). *Children, the environment and accidents.* Pitman Medical Publishing, London.

Kritzinger, E. E. *Differential diagnosis of the red eye.* Smith and Nephew Pharmaceuticals Ltd, Romford.

Levene, G. M. and Calnan, C. D. (1974). *A colour atlas of dermatology.* Wolfe Medical Publications, London.

Manson, P. (1982). *Tropical diseases* (18th edn). Bailliere Tindall, Eastbourne.

Matthew, H. and Lawson, A. A. H. (1979). *Treatment of common acute poisonings* (4th edn). Churchill Livingstone, Edinburgh.

McGregor, I. A. (1980). *Fundamental techniques of plastic surgery and their surgical applications* (7th edn). Churchill Livingstone, Edinburgh.

McRae, R. (1981). *Practical fracture treatment.* Churchill Livingstone, Edinburgh. In my opinion, the best book on fractures for the casualty officer.

Monthly index of medical specialities (MIMS). Medical Publications Ltd, London. Published monthly.

Owen-Smith, M. S. (1981). *High velocity missile wounds.* Arnold, London.

Potter, J. M. (1984). *The practical management of head injuries* (4th edn). Lloyd-Luke, London. Contains the best summary of eye signs in head injuries; useful in general too.

Proudfoot, A. T. (1982). *Diagnosis and management of acute poisoning.* Blackwell Scientific Publications, Oxford.

Rains, A. J. H. and Ritchie, H. D. (eds) (1984). *Bailey and Love's short practice of surgery* (19th edn). Lewis,

London.

Richards, A. B. *Ocular emergencies*. Smith and Nephew Pharmaceuticals Ltd, Welwyn Garden City. Elementary and clearly illustrated.

Robertson, C. and Little, K. (eds) (1983). *A manual of accident and emergency resuscitation*. Wiley, Chichester.

Semple, C. (1979). *The primary management of hand injuries*. Pitman Medical Publishing, London.

Settle, J. A. D. *Burns: the first 48 hours*. Smith and Nephew Pharmaceuticals Ltd, Romford. Excellent.

Snook, R. (1974). *Medical aid at accidents*. Update, London. Definitive for ambulance and fire service crews; useful for surgical flying squads.

Transport emergency cards (1986). Chemical Industries Association Ltd, Kings Buildings, Smith Square, London SW1P 3JJ. Important source book of toxic lorry freights. Chem-safe manual (supplied free) tells you how to get assistance. All A & E departments should have this work of reference.

Vale, J. A. and Meredith, T. J. (1980). *Poisoning: diagnosis and treatment*. Update, London. Not a complete guide, but of a high standard and very well presented.

Valman, H. B. (1979). *Accident and emergency paediatrics* (2nd edn). Blackwell Scientific Publications, Oxford.

Warwick, R. and Williams, P. L. (eds) (1980). *Gray's anatomy* (36th edn). Churchill Livingstone, Edinburgh. The basis of the treatment of trauma.

Weatherall, D. J. (ed.) (1987). *Oxford textbook of medicine* (2nd edn). Oxford University Press.

Wood, B. (ed.) (1982). *A paediatric vade-mecum* (10th edn). Lloyd-Luke, London. A great comfort in times of doubt with simple tables of drugs, treatments, and dosages; well indexed.

Yates, D. W. and Redmond, A. D. (1985). *Lecture notes on accident and emergency medicine*. Blackwell Scientific Publications, Oxford.

Index

Main headings are shown in CAPITALS. Headings are immediately followed by the principal page reference(s); other references to the same subject follow, after a semi-colon.